D1305808

Modeling

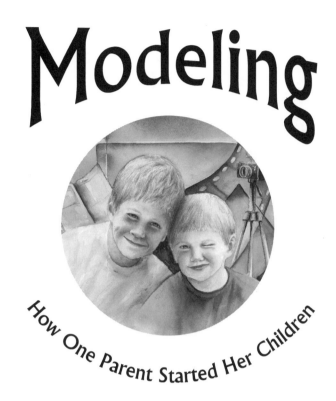

How One Parent Started Her Children

Susan M. Halter

BELIEVE IN YOURSELF
PUBLISHING CO.
Spring Lake, Michigan

BELIEVE IN YOURSELF PUBLISHING
7133 14th Street
Spring Lake, Michigan 49415

Publisher's Cataloging-in-Publication Data
Halter, Susan, M.
      Modeling: how one parent started her children /
      Susan M. Halter – Spring Lake, Mich.:
      Believe In Yourself Publishing, 1998.
            p. ill. cm.

      ISBN 0-9659634-8-9
      1. Careers – Juvenile. 2. Young Adult – Entertainment.
      3. Entertainment Business – Minors. I Title.
LCCN 97-94557   1998

02 01 00 99 ✳ 5 4 3 2 1

Printed in United States

To my sons, Jason Roy Randal Halter and Nicholas James Edward Halter, who are my inspiration; to my husband, Randal E. Halter, without whom I would not be who I am today; to my sister Rosalie and her family for always being there for me; and to the author, yes, that's me, who has learned that if you believe, you can achieve.

Last of all, to my mom who passed away before the completion of this book and is dearly missed. Thank you, Mom, for your smiles, your encouragement and for giving me my life. Thank you, Mom, for believing in me.

Contents

Preface

My sons, Jason (12) and Nicholas (10), have appeared in commercials videos, and print advertisements since they were babies. Many parents, fascinated by what we do, have asked me for advice about how to start their children in the modeling and commercial business and what to expect. I tell them that this field is like a magnet: It pulls you in without your knowing what you are getting yourself into. Erroneous, misleading advice is plentiful, but honest hands-on experience is scarce. To my knowledge, no tested resource on this topic exists which explains, from a parent's perspective, how and where to begin, what pitfalls to avoid, and how to stay sane in unexpected situations.

Modeling: How One Parent Started Her Children combines my personal experience, observation, and research. I take readers, step by step, through the process of deciding whether modeling would be good for their children and could fit into their lifestyle; finding and evaluating agencies to represent them; preparing an inexpensive but effective portfolio; anticipating and surviving the first audition; and doing well at the first and subsequent jobs. I also advise parents on how to guide the careers of their children while allowing them to have a secure, normal childhood. And I include numerous samples of actual paperwork related to the industry as well as a helpful glossary to identify terms for the uninitiated. My goal is to help parents and their children benefit from my family's years of experience and success in the field.

FROM THE PUBLISHER

This book is designed by the author to share her personal experiences with regard to the subject matter. It is not the purpose of this volume to be an exhaustive compilation of already existing texts, but to compliment and amplify aspects of other available materials. The author intends not only to educate her readers, but also to entertain them.

Anyone planning to enter the modeling field must expect to invest much time and effort, with no guarantees of success. This volume cannot be a substitute for the necessary hard work, and the "breaks" that are needed to forge a successful career.

While the author and publisher have made every effort to make this book as complete and accurate as possible, it is acknowledged that there may be mistakes in both the typographical and content nature and other possible types of errors. Therefore, neither the author nor the publisher shall have any liability or responsibility to any person or entity with respect to any loss or damage caused or alleged to be caused directly or indirectly by the information contained in this work.

Believe in Yourself Publishing Co.
May 1998

Acknowledgments

I gratefully acknowledge the following people and organizations for granting me permission to reprint their material in this book:

Susan Garvey, *react Magazine*, Advance Magazine Publication, Inc., 711 Third Avenue, New York, NY 10017: Article excerpts from "Her Own Person," by Jacqueline Austin, copyright 1996;

Gary Marsh, Breakdown Services, LTD, *C/D Directory*, P.O. Box 69277, Los Angeles, CA 90069;

McDonald's Corporation, 2010 E. Higgins Road, Elk Grove Village, Illinois 60007: "Tips for Actors and Actresses Working in McDonald's Video Programs," Video 25— "Heroism";

Harry Medved, Screen Actors Guild National Headquarters, 5757 Wilshire Blvd., Los Angeles, CA 90036-3600: "Screen Actors Guild Branch Offices Listing"; "Screen Actors Guild New Membership Information"; "Screen Actors Guild Fact Sheet Regarding Talent Agencies"; "SAG Advice Regarding Agents"; "What All Performers Should Know About AFTRA-SAG . . . and the 'Business'"; "Acting In Your Interest"; "Profile—Screen Actors Guild";

Johnathan Miller, Television Index, Inc., 40-29 27th Street, Long Island City, New York 11101: *Ross Reports Television*, March 95, "TV Pro-Log Digest Television Program and Production News"; Subscription page of "Services and Publications";

Ray Greene, Editor-in-Chief, *BOXOFFICE* Magazine, 6640 Sunset Blvd., Suite 100, Hollywood, CA 90028: Excerpts from "Sneak Preview" section titled "Ghost of a Chance," by Christine James, April 1995; and from "Sneak Preview" section titled "A Family 'Tie," by Kim Williamson, June 1995;

Suzanne Harper, Executive Editor, Disney Adventures, 114 Fifth Avenue, 16th Floor, New York, NY 10011-5690: Excerpts from "Kids" by Liz Smith, March 1996.

And I thank each of the following people for playing an important part in the success of this book:

LeeAnn Frame, for her creative artwork and design for the cover of this book.

Nancy O'Neill, for coming into my life at the right time and believing in me.

Monica Archer, for providing continued support for this project and the energy to motivate me one step further, to just go for it.

Modeling

CHAPTER 1

"Proceed with Caution" When Entering the Modeling Industry

Probably, like many other parents, at some point you look at your new baby or young child and think how gorgeous he or she is, just as cute and cuddly as all those babies and children on television and in magazines. But watch out—some people know how vulnerable we are. A caution flag should go up in your mind when you hear radio advertisement about searches for new faces; or see newspaper ads that may begin with "MODELS," which in the past have been listed under "Help Wanted" in my area; or receive an agency postcard or letter that comes addressed "To the Parents of . . . " Companies which advertise in these ways probably are not the type of company you are looking for. Some of them charge exhorbitant fees, often hundreds of dollars, for a brief photo session or a one- or two-day "convention," neither of which is likely to lead anywhere for most people. Others will come to your home and give you a great sales pitch but very little solid information about the modeling and commercial industry. I speak from experience. I was one of those naive parents who was fooled into writing several checks in the beginning. Fortunately, I sensed I was making a mistake before the first check cleared. I learned a lot from my mistake, and so can you. Before you release large sums of your hard-earned money, read on. You have in your hands the information I wish I had had when I started my son Jason in commercial work.

Promotional or Management Companies

People often ask me about my children's modeling career. The first question they ask is usually the same; "How did you get started?" The second is, "How did you find the agencies that don't charge fees?" What attracted me to this industry in the beginning (1985) was a postcard about modeling I received in the mail and letters from different companies telling me that they could promote my son.

I called one of the companies and agreed to have a representative visit me at home. She showed me books with pictures of other children who had signed with her company and who now, supposedly, were successful. As part of the interview process, the agency representative asked to carry my infant son Jason, saying that if he cried, the interview would be over and the agency could not accept him. But of course he did not cry, because most four-to-five-month-old babies usually do not experience separation anxiety yet. So, he was acceptable, a perfect model baby. I was so excited! My son had a chance to be in a commercial, a rare chance, only 1.7 percent, the representative told me, but I thought, none at all if I didn't sign.

She made it sound too easy: "You don't have to pay us all at one time." It was suggested that I post-date several checks for the amounts requested and the agency would hold the checks in its vault and only cash each check as the date became current. I wrote a check for fifty dollars that day and also wrote five more checks, four for fifty dollars and the last one for seventy-five, one for each of the following five months. I did what so many others do: I fell for the sales pitch. The interview was over and I was told that I would be notified of a time and a place for Jason to have his picture taken for the agency's files.

I was so naive! Not being able to sleep well that night, and fearing that I had made a bad decision, I went to my bank the next morning and stopped payment on the check I had written the day before. Then I took advantage of the agency's cancellation period to notify the staff of my intention to cancel everything so they would send my checks back, and they did—but not before depositing the current fifty-dollar check. Thank goodness I had put a stop payment on it. I was still curious about agency's motives and decided to investigate further.

Now it was time to do my homework and think of people who might be able to shed some light on this subject and guide me in the right direction. Before my first son was born, I had been a professional cheerleader for the United States Football League, Chicago Franchise, The Chicago Blitz. Having also worked in the marketing and promotional department of the franchise, I had at least a direction in which to start. I called my knowledgeable former supervisor, and asked about agencies that would charge an advance fee in order to help find work for my son in commercials. He responded emphatically: "You do not have to pay anyone up front to promote your children in the modeling or acting field! The choice is yours," he explained, "but you can do the same thing they are doing—contact the talent agencies yourself. You don't need a management agency or any kind of company that wants to take money out of your pocket up front before you even receive your first job."

At the time, I did not realize there is a difference between a modeling agency and a management agency; I assumed the people contacting me represented modeling, talent, or casting agencies. But they did not; they represented "management" or "promotional companies," which are supposed to send your pictures to people in the commercial industry and help you find work. Whether these companies indeed do so, is something one should verify. In contrast, a talent agency franchised with the Screen Actors Guild (SAG) <u>does not take your money in advance</u> (or let's say it certainly should not). If a franchised agency does, SAG wants to hear about it. *A legitimate talent agency is not paid until the talent is paid from a booked job,* which makes sense and gives the agency a reason to promote you. In Chapter Two, you will find the information you need to help you locate and choose talent agencies.

Seminars and Conventions—Be Careful!

You should be cautious regarding the one- or two-day talent-search seminars which are usually advertised either on the radio or in newspapers. Although I have not attended one of these myself, a friend of my brother did. Unfortunately, the friend did not know I was knowledgeable about the business until after he had surrendered his full payment. After talking to me, my brother's friend said he wished he had had a resource like this book, before he had fallen for the sales pitch of the seminar ad. He was willing to share his experience with me, so that I could caution others not to be gullible.

Typically, you might attend a free modeling or talent search meeting, then receive an invitation to preregister for a convention, for which there is a charge. You must pay a portion of the fee by a certain date with a certified check or money order only; personal checks are usually not accepted (maybe because it is too easy to stop payment on them). You have spent money right from the beginning, but what if you are sick and cannot go? After reading through all the information more than once, I did not find a way to receive your deposit money back if you cannot attend. Always read the fine print before you pay for services, to make sure there is a way out if you still choose to attend one of these conventions. A telephone call to the company's main office can help you find out how to receive your deposit back if the paperwork does not explain how to retrieve it. You may be surprised by what you are told—I was!

On the day of the convention, you must pay the difference owed in cash or by certified check or money order. These charges might be over two-hundred dollars for an adult and over three-hundred for an adult with a child; in the latter case, that's because you have to pay two fees, one for the child and one for the person accompanying the child! Six- to seven-hundred people were at the seminar my brother's friend attended. The information provided was so general and limited in each category presented, that it was hard to grasp the reality of the business, especially for a beginner. At the end of the convention, he was given very little information to take home regarding local agencies he could contact on his own, since he was not chosen for the convention callbacks—not even a telephone number. And that was it. He was now out over two-hundred dollars and had very little to show for it!

While writing this book, I could not pass up the opportunity to attend one of the advertised talent searches myself. Remember the ads I referred to earlier, which appear in my local newspaper, with the heading "MODELS"? Well, this time I traveled to the free interview being offered at a local meeting center. I had personal experience with the house calls, my brother's friend's information about the convention he attended, and now another potential first-hand experience to share with my readers.

There appeared to be more than two-hundred adults with small children attending the first of two sessions scheduled on the same night. A fast-talking, don't-let-anyone-get-a-word-in-edgewise representative came into the conference room late, introduced herself, and gave the crowd a little background about the company and the few people it was responsible for promoting. She stated several times that the company could not guarantee assignments for anyone at any time if he or she were chosen to come back for a photo session. I'll give her credit for that admission. However, as the representative went on to explain, the printed sheet of information that we were given after the video interview did say, "We do guarantee the necessary promotion and exposure needed to land potential modeling or acting assignments." (Now, remember what you just read; you will find it interesting later, as I did.)

We were told several times not to be disappointed if we were not chosen to come back for the photo session; "It does not mean you are ugly," it just means you are probably not what the advertisers are looking for at this time. Doesn't that sound as if a person has to be chosen to come back for the photo session in order to be represented by this company? It does to me, especially since the information sheet stated that the selection process was based on "personality, attitude, photogenic look, and ability to take directions." Oddly, we had to call the next day an out-of-state long-distance number (why not back at the same meeting establishment?) to see if we were selected for the photo session.

But the best part was saved for the end. The fee! It was over one-hundred fifty dollars, which was to pay for a one-roll-of-film photo session, and a handful of small prints for the model, one of which was to go on the company headsheet, like the one on display and was to be sent to advertising agencies within a certain range of where the model lived and to agencies in New York City. A headsheet could be several portrait-like photos grouped on one poster. Payment had to be made at the photo session by charge card, cashier's check, or money order. A personal check would only be accepted with a cash or charge card deposit. I started to become suspicious when we were told that questions were to not to be asked, and that we should hold our questions until it was our turn to be interviewed while the video camera was taping. This was not turning out the way I hoped. Why wouldn't they have an open forum for questions?

The next day, I called the telephone number on the sheet we had received, to give this company one last chance to prove itself worthy of its fee. I asked for the names of a couple of the advertising agencies to which the company representatives send the headsheet, to verify that they do what they claimed. After being told by the first person I spoke to that my request was impractical (she said they could not give out names or everyone would be calling those people, and the advertising companies would be angry—which makes sense), I asked for just one name. I was put on hold for several minutes; a second person picked up the phone, then a third person. I told the third person, "People around me think this is money thrown out the window. Will you please give me one, just one name I can call to verify that you send out the headsheet you claim you send?"

The person still refused. He avoided the question by telling me, "You know, if you have your own composite or professional pictures of yourself, you can send them directly to us." He also said that I did not have to go to the photo session and pay the fee. That fee was just for people who needed to have their photo taken. Thinking I had heard him wrong, I asked him to repeat himself. I hadn't. He said the same thing. "Why didn't the person in charge that evening tell us that?" I asked. "Plus, that is not how it's stated in the paperwork I received last night," I added. I even read to him a few lines from the paper I had in front of me. With that, he cut the conversation short and told me he did not feel like wasting his time on the phone with me any longer. I added once again that I had wanted to see if the company was willing to give me one agency name to back up their claims. "I guess I'll have to draw my own conclusion," I said. "Well, I guess so. You are entitled to that," he answered. End of conversation! Refer back to where I said they put in print that they DO guarantee the necessary promotion and so on. Why wouldn't they demostrate how they guarantee their work? They could not, or perhaps chose not to, or prove to me that they would actively promote their talent.

This is what we are up against when we want to start in modeling, and there seems to be no where else to find information unless we know someone in the business who can guide us. No wonder so many people sign. We would love to see our kids on television reaching for opportunities, so we decide to go for it, only to be disappointed in the end.

Nevertheless, choosing whether to go to these meetings or conventions or having a home meeting is always left up to the individual. I cannot tell you what your decision should be, but I encourage you to be careful and to ask questions. As the old saying goes, "If it sounds to good to be true, it probably is." I am hoping this book will guide you toward the goal you would like to pursue for your children or even perhaps for yourself while helping you avoid the pitfalls of this industry. Please write and let me know how you fare.

CHAPTER 2

Agencies: How to Locate and Work with Them

Selecting Agencies

What better place to start than the Screen Actors Guild (SAG). Yes, the same union that the Hollywood stars belong to. After finding the number for my local branch of Screen Actors Guild, I called for information. I was told to send a self-addressed, stamped envelope and a letter asking for a list of all modeling agencies registered with that branch. If an agency were SAG franchised, I thought, it was probably legitimate.

Before receiving my list from SAG, my sister-in-law gave me a number of a friend's daughter who was a model registered with a talent agency in downtown Chicago. Since she was happy with that agency, I asked her for the name and address, so that when I started my selection process, I could contact that agency. Having a contact name at the agency helps, too. She also suggested contacting several agencies at one time to save time. During our conversation I had asked if any of these agencies want money up front for any reason for either photos or to register. Her response was,"No way, and to steer clear from any that ever might." Living in the Chicago area at the time, I had many agencies from which to choose. (I was spoiled! Five years later, when I moved to Michigan, I found only one agency within an hour's drive that was SAG franchised.) The area in which you live could have a great effect on the availability of agencies and work. In my opinion, if you live in or near one of the regional Screen Actors Guild offices, your chances of staying actively involved in this business are greater than if you live more than a few hours away. There are just more choices of agencies in the bigger cities.

After I had selected my first five agencies, I called to see if they listed (represented) children, because the information I had received from them did not always specify age groups. Some agencies do not accept anyone under age four or two, etc., or even accept children at all. Some like to set up an interview; others tell you the days and hours they are open to walk-ins, which means you do not need an interview appointment to stop by and drop off snapshots and introduce yourself and your child. However, agency staff members do not appreciate it if you just happen to be in the neighborhood and stop in at anytime.

Most agencies I have worked with, tightly schedule their days. Wanting to help me succeed, Shirley Hamilton, a top talent agent in Chicago and a wonderful person, once told me, "Obey the rules!" It's good to follow her advice, especially in the beginning; once the agents know you, conditions might change, but still have consideration, no matter how popular your children become.

I had my list of agencies to send my sons photo's, to see if they would accept Jason, and their registration procedures. It was now time for me to send photos. Most agencies want you to send them your own photographs, just a few for now. Professional photos or composites are not necessary for the first contact and might not be until your children are older. So save your money!

Since I had chosen five different agencies I would be sending five-to-ten snapshots of Jason to each. Being a new parent, I always had my camera within arm's reach and took dozens of my own pictures, capturing different moods, expressions, and activities, mostly close-up. I was not going to spend a great deal of money in the beginning for professional pictures when I did not know whether any of the agencies would agree to register my son. And I am glad I did not, because snapshots are indeed all they wanted; a young child changes much too fast to justify spending a lot of money on professional photos.

Here is my checklist for what to assemble for each agency; 1) the photographs, with personal information, such as name, address, etc. on the back (for detailed instructions about what information to include on photographs, see Chapter Three); 2) a sturdy envelope, with adequate postage, addressed to the agency and a contact name if you have one; 3) Send certified mail with "Return Receipt Requested", if you want to know exactly when and whom received your photos at the agency; 4) a self-addressed, stamped envelope to hasten the agency's

Nicholas and Jason Halter Snapshots

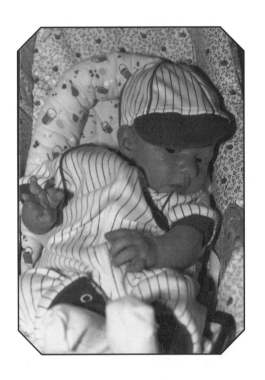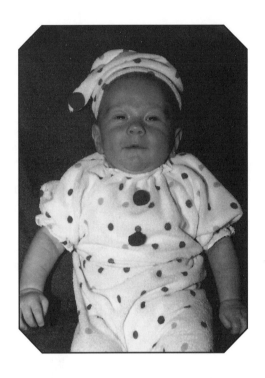

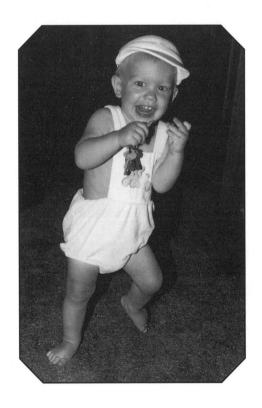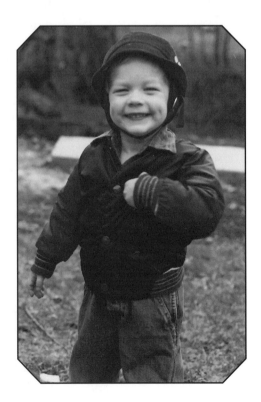

response—rejection or acceptance—to you. Some agencies will send back photos if they do not accept your children but not many. Or you may receive a "thank you but no thank you" letter.

After sending my packets of snapshots to the five agencies, all I could do was wait. Notification might take a week or months, you just never know. It is not a good idea to call the agencies you have sent pictures to and ask if they have received them, although your patience will be tested. I did call and only one agency representative took the time to see if my packet had arrived. I can now understand why they say, "Don't call us, we'll call you." Agencies receive so many pictures of talent wanting to register with them that it is almost impossible for agency personnel to know if they have received yours yet. This is another reason why legitimate talent agencies do not take your money up front. More people than they can accept send pictures and want to be registered; therefore, they do not have to advertise in the newspapers or on the radio for talent.

Don't be surprised if, after you are registered with the talent agency and feel pretty comfortable with the person who is handling the children's department, that person leaves. One exception is Toni Wilson from the Shirley Hamilton Agency, who has continued to be with Shirley Hamilton since the day we registered with them. I have noticed over the years that some agencies seem to go through a house cleaning of sorts every two years or so, which means that new employees come in, and gone are the ones you are used to and who know you. With new employees in an agency, it is like starting all over again with that agency. The changes discouraged me at first, but then I accepted them as another challenge. As with anything else, if you want to be successful at what you do, you must be persistent and overcome obstacles along the way.

Obtaining SAG Lists

To save you time, I have included a list of the Screen Actors Guild (SAG) branch offices, starting with the National Headquarters in Los Angeles. Just like any business, from time to time they might move from one location to another, so when contacting one of these branch offices to obtain a current list of talent agencies in your area or throughtout the United States, do call to make sure it is still located at the same address. For instance, when I first started in this business the national headquarters for SAG was located in Hollywood, CA. While updating my own list this year, I realized the headquarters had been moved to Los Angeles. Making a simple phone call saved me postage and a further delay in obtaining my information if the forwarding address had expired.

The California and New York Screen Actors Guild offices have a monthly updated list of more than five-hundred talent agencies registered with SAG throughout the United States. A small fee of one-to-three dollars might be charged for this list. Write to the branch office (see list) closest to your hometown and request their latest SAG Talent Agents list. Due to the monthly updating by the Screen Actor Guild staff, it would of been impossible to list all the agencies in this book and have the list current. The branch offices should be able to give you a list of agencies in their region. Some will also send you the list covering the entire United States, as do the California and New York offices. But, again, call to make sure the SAG office in your area is still at the same address, and ask if there is a charge for their lists and which ones are available. To expedite your order, send a self-addressed stamped envelope.

When you receive your lists, note the abbreviations, if any, which usually are located after the telephone numbers on the SAG Talent Agents list. They tell you what type of work the agents offer, e.g.; (T) Theater/Television; (C) commercials; (FS) Full Service; (Y) Young Performers; (A) Adults. I am very pleased that the Screen Actors Guild has granted me permission to reprint so much of their helpful information throughout this book.

In Chapter Six, which talks about "Self-Promoting," I have gathered valuable information about how to obtain lists of casting agencies that are members of the Casting Society of America. Casting agencies differ from talent agencies, you should also send them photos, so that casting agents know which talent agencies represent your children should they wish to have them audition. Casting agency lists are difficult to obtain because you and I, as the talent, do not deal directly with them; the talent agent does. There is one exception, but you must follow the rules when contacting them. Please read Chapter Six before you do anything regarding the casting agents. The chapter on Self-Promoting also includes names and addresses of popular television shows, and the people who are responsible for casting that you may want to send photos to in addition to the talent agencies.

★ BRANCH OFFICES ★

NATIONAL HEADQUARTERS
5757 Wilshire Boulevard
Los Angeles, CA 90036-3600
(213) 954-1600

ARIZONA 1616 E Indian School Rd
#330
Phoenix, AZ 85016
(602) 265-2712

ATLANTA 455 E Paces Ferry Rd NE
Suite #334
Atlanta, GA 30305
(404) 239-0131

BOSTON 11 Beacon St
#512
Boston, MA 02108
(617) 742-2688

CHICAGO 1 E Erie Dr
Suite 650
Chicago, IL 60611
(312)573-8081

CLEVELAND*1030 Euclid Ave
Suite #429
Cleveland, OH 44115
(216) 579-9305

DALLAS 6060 N Central Expy
#302/LB 604
Dallas, TX 75206
(214) 363-8300

DENVER** 950 S Cherry St #502
Denver, CO 80222
(303) 757-6226

DETROIT 28690 Southfield Rd
Suite 290 A & B
Lathrup Vlg, MI 48076
(810) 559-9540

FLORIDA*** 7300 N Kendall Dr
Suite #620
Miami, FL 33156-7840
(305) 670-7677

CENTRAL 646 W Colonial Dr
FLORIDA Orlando, FL 32804
(407) 649-3100

HAWAII 949 Kapiolani Bl
#105
Honolulu, HI 96814
(808) 596-0388

HOUSTON 2650 Fountainview Dr
#326
Houston, TX 77057
(713) 972-1806

MINNEAPOLIS/ 708 N 1st St
ST. PAUL* Suite #343A
Minneapolis, MN 55401
(612) 371-9120

NASHVILLE 1108 17th Ave S
Nashville, TN 37212
(615) 327-2944

NEVADA 3900 Paradise Rd
#206
Las Vegas, NV 89109
(702) 737-8818

NEW YORK 1515 Broadway
44th Fl
New York, NY 10036
(212) 944-1030

NORTH CAROLINA 321 N Front St
Wilmington NC 28401
(910) 762-1889

PHILADELPHIA 230 S Broad St
Suite 500
Philadelphia, PA 19102
(215) 545-3150

PORTLAND 3030 SW Moody
#104
Portland OR 97201
(503) 279-9600

ST. LOUIS* 906 Olive St
#1006
St Louis, MO 63101
(314) 231-8410

SAN DIEGO 7827 Convoy Ct
#400
San Diego, CA 92111
(619) 278-7695

SAN FRANCISCO 235 Pine St
11th Fl
San Francisco, CA 94104
(415) 391-7510

SEATTLE 601 Valley St
#100
Seattle, WA 98109
(206) 282-2506

WASHINGTON/ 4340 E West Hwy
BALTIMORE Suite #204
Bethesda, MD 20814
(301) 657-2560

* AFTRA offices which also handle SAG business for their areas.
** Denver is a regional office which also covers New Mexico & Utah.
*** Florida is a regional office which also covers Alabama, Arkansas, Louisiana,
Mississippi, West Virginia, U.S. Virgin Islands, Puerto Rico and the Caribbean.

★ DUES ★

SAG dues are based on SAG earnings, and are billed twice each year.
Each SAG member will pay basic annual dues of $85.00. In addition, those members earning more than $5,000.00 per year under SAG contracts will pay 1 ½% of such income in excess of $5,000 to a maximum of $150,000. Members who are paying full dues to another performers' union and earn less than $25,000 per year under SAG contracts will receive a reduction of $10.00 per year. Members whose SAG earnings exceed $25,000 per year will pay full dues, regardless of other guild affiliations.

FACT SHEET REGARDING
TALENT AGENCIES

(The following information is being distributed by the Los Angeles Office of the Consumer Protection Division of the Federal Trade Commission:)

Question: What is the difference between a legitimate talent agency and one whose purpose is to separate you from your money?

Answer: The legitimate talent agency does not charge a fee payable in advance for registering you, for resumes, for public relations services, for screen tests, for photographs, for acting lessons, or for many other services used to separate you from your money. If you are signed as a client by a legitimate talent agency, you will pay such agency nothing until you work and then 10 percent of your earnings as a performer -- but nothing in advance. Legitimate talent agencies normally do not advertise for clients in newspaper classified columns nor do they solicit through the mail.

Question: Are legitimate talent agencies licensed by the State of California?

Answer: Yes. Such talent agencies are licensed by the State as Talent Agents and most established agencies in the motion picture and television film field are also franchised by the Screen Actors Guild. You should be extremely careful of any talent agency not licensed by the State.

Question: What about personal managers and business managers?

Answer: There are well established firms in the business of personal management and business management but such firms in the main handle established artists and they do not advertise for newcomers, nor promise employment.

Question: What about photographers?

Answer: If a purported talent agent seeks to send you to a particular photographer for pictures, what should you do? Hold your wallet tight and run for the nearest exit. Chances are he's phony and he makes his money by splitting the photographer's fee. If you need photographers, choose your own photographer. Better still, try another agent. But don't pay anything in advance.

SAG ADVICE
REGARDING AGENTS

1. Make sure your agent is franchised with SAG before signing an agency contract or accepting verbal representation.

2. Agent's clients lists are available to SAG members for inspection at the SAG's Agency Department.

3. All changes in your SAG agency listing must be made in writing - we cannot accept them by phone. Always include your Social Security number.

4. "Verbal" contracts (where their is no written agency contract in existence, or while new contracts are being prepared) can be filed with SAG by the performer sending SAG a written letter stating that they are represented by XYZ talent agent for XYZ field of representation; or by the Talent Agent using the Client Confirmation Form. This information will remain in SAG's computer system until we are advised, in writing, to remove and/or change such information.

5. Improper behavior by an agent should be reported to SAG immediately. These matters are handled confidentially. Your name is never used without your consent.

6. SAG does not have jurisdiction over print work and/or modeling.

7. With respect to all moneys for TV and Theatrical compensation, the agent has three (3) business days from the time the agency receives the money; and with respect to moneys received as compensation for television commercials, five (5) business days from the time the agent receives the money from the employer. Commencing November 21, 1990, payments received from an employer drawn on a financial institution located in a state other than the state in which the agent's office is located, the time for the agent to pay over to the actor shall be extended to seven (7) calendar days.

8. Make sure that you are using the SAG form contract when signing with an agency, and never sign contracts that contain blank spaces or are missing information.

9. SAG does not regulate Personal Managers.

The First Contact by an Agency

After weeks of waiting and becoming discouraged because I had heard nothing, I received my first response; a postcard from one of the agencies I had sent photos to, with instructions about how to proceed (see insert). I was told to send more photographs with the same information on the back as before, and to continue doing so every six months to update its files, and to include a self-addressed, stamped envelope so the agency could send me information regarding a work permit. You read it correctly, a work permit! Even at nine months old, my son had to have a work permit. I followed those instructions, and a week later I had all the necessary information back from the agency. I also received positive responses from the other talent agencies, along with all their paperwork. Some agencies include all the necessary information when they first contact you. You can see from the examples, that each agency has different paperwork requirements. Be prepared for negative responses, but do not be discouraged from contacting more agencies. (See sample Letters of Intent, etc.)

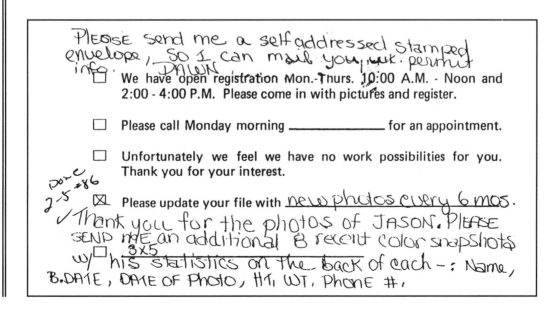

15

Z 103 795 269

**Receipt for
Certified Mail**

No Insurance Coverage Provided
Do not use for International Mail
(See Reverse)

UNITED STATES
POSTAL SERVICE

Sent to	
Street and No.	
P.O., State and ZIP Code	
Postage	$
Certified Fee	
Special Delivery Fee	
Restricted Delivery Fee	
Return Receipt Showing to Whom & Date Delivered	
Return Receipt Showing to Whom, Date, and Addressee's Address	
TOTAL Postage & Fees	$
Postmark or Date	

PS Form **3800,** March 1993

Fold at line over top of envelope to the
right of the return address

CERTIFIED

Z 103 795 269

MAIL

Is your **RETURN ADDRESS** completed on the reverse side?

SENDER:
- Complete items 1 and/or 2 for additional services.
- Complete items 3, 4a, and 4b.
- Print your name and address on the reverse of this form so that we can return this card to you.
- Attach this form to the front of the mailpiece, or on the back if space does not permit.
- Write *"Return Receipt Requested"* on the mailpiece below the article number.
- The Return Receipt will show to whom the article was delivered and the date delivered.

I also wish to receive the following services (for an extra fee):

1. ☐ Addressee's Address
2. ☐ Restricted Delivery

Consult postmaster for fee.

3. Article Addressed to:	4a. Article Number
	4b. Service Type
	☐ Registered ☐ Certified
	☐ Express Mail ☐ Insured
	☐ Return Receipt for Merchandise ☐ COD
	7. Date of Delivery
5. Received By: *(Print Name)*	8. Addressee's Address *(Only if requested and fee is paid)*
6. Signature: *(Addressee or Agent)* X	

Thank you for using Return Receipt Service.

PS Form **3811,** December 1994

Domestic Return Receipt

16

Talent Agency

LETTER OF INTENT

This agency intends to seek employment for the following minor:

Jason Halter

This is in compliance with the Federal Child Labor Laws
(as provided by the Fair Labor Standards Act - Section 3,
52 Stat. 1060, as amended: 29 U.S.C. 203)

Sincerely,

Explanation Letter from Talent Agencies

Client   (708)
Talent - (708)

DEAR PARENTS,

IT IS ESSENTIAL FOR US TO HAVE A WORK PERMIT FOR YOUR CHILD BEFORE WE SEND HIM OR HER OUT ON AN AUDITION. CHILDREN WILL NOT BE BOOKED UNLESS WE HAVE A WORK PERMIT IN THEIR FILE.

ENCLOSED IS A LETTER OF INTENT WHICH YOU WILL NEED IN ORDER TO OBTAIN THE WORK PERMIT FOR YOUR CHILD.

PLEASE GO TO YOUR LOCAL BOARD OF EDUCATION AND OBTAIN ONE AS SOON AS POSSIBLE.

THE LETTER OF INTENT IS FROM   TALENT WHICH IS THE AGENCY THAT IS GOING TO TRY TO OBTAIN WORK FOR YOUR CHILD.

WHEN YOU RECEIVE THE WORK PERMIT PLEASE SEND US A COPY AND KEEP THE ORIGINAL WITH YOU WHEN YOU HAVE A BOOKING FROM US. SHOW THE ORIGINAL TO THE PERSONS IN CHARGE OF THE SHOOT.

THANK YOU,

PRESIDENT

SOME SCHOOLS THAT ISSUE WORK PERMITS ARE ON THE ATTACHED LIST. IF YOU ARE NOT IN THOSE DISTRICTS PLEASE GO TO YOUR LOCAL BOARD OF EDUCATION:

Client - (708)
Talent - (708)

LETTER OF INTENT

The undersigned agency owner intends to attempt to secure employment for the model, _____, a minor, in conformity with the requirements of Section 24 of the Rules and Regulations of the Illinois Child Labor Law, Ch. 48, Ill. Rev. Stat., 31.3, et seq. which states:

Children under the age of 16 have specific restrictions with respect to the number of hours which they can work in a given day and/or week. A summary of the restrictions which apply between Memorial Day and Labor Day as set forth in the Illinois Department of Labor's Child Labor Regulations are as follows:*

1. Minors under 8 years of age may not be employed, used or exhibited as a model for more than 2 hours in any one day nor than 10 hours in any one week.

2. Minors between the ages of 8 and 13 years of age may not be employed for:

   (a) More than 4 hours in any one day in which school is not in session;
   (b) More than 20 hours during any week in which school is not in session for at least 3 days.

3. Children between the ages of 14 and 16 cannot work more than 8 hours on any day or more than 48 hours in any week.

4. Children can work only between the hours of 7 a.m. and 9 p.m. during the summer months (i.e., period between Memorial Day and Labor Day).

*Stricter rules apply during the school year.

In addition, we confirm that this child is age _____ to date
_____.
          (Today's Date)

The child mentioned above with the consent and support of the parents and the representing agency, M/A   Talent, agrees to follow the code of the Illinois Child Labor Law concerning the number of hours and days in accordance to the age of this child as stated above.

_____
                    (Agency Owner)

<u>LETTER OF INTENT</u>

DATE: _12-01-91_

To the City or County Superintendent of Schools:

The undersigned intends to place the child applying for this certificate, _Jason Roy Raulel Halter_, who is _6_ years old, as a model/actor for not more than or for any period in excess of that permitted by Illinois Statute.

Thank you,

Susan M. Halter
Signature of Parent

Children under 7 years old may work for not more than two hours in any one day, nor more than ten hours in any one week.

Children 8-13 years old may work for not more than three hours in any one day in which school is in session, or more than four hours in any other day; or more than eighteen hours/week in which school is in session for more than three days, or more than twenty hours/week in any other week.

Children 14 & 15 years old may work for not more than 6 consecutive days in any one week or more than 8 hours in any one day. Children may not work between 7:00pm and 7:00am except from June 1st until Labor Day. School age children may not work more than 3 hours a day when school is in session, nor may the combined hours of work and school exceed 8 hours a day.

20

We have received and reviewed the photos submitted to our office. Since we are booked with interviews for several months and we would like to have you registered with our agency, I have enclosed our registration card. Please fill the card out completely and return it to our office along with 20 more photos . Be sure to put your complete address on the card. We have also enclosed an letter of intent for a work permit for your child.

We will then file your photos so that we have them available to send to clients requesting photos of talents in your catagory.

If after one year, you do not receive a booking from our office; please update the stats with us so that we keep your childs photos in the active file.

Thank you for a quick response.

Sincerely.

Registration Card

Date _____ T/I File No. _____ Male ___ Female ___   Birthdate_____

Child_____ SS#_____
     (Last Name),   (First Name)

Address_____ Home Phone: _____

City_____ State_____ Zip_____ Alt Phone: _____

Mother's Name_____ WORK # _____ Hair Color _____

Father's Name_____ WORK # _____ Eye Color _____

DATE   HEIGHT   WEIGHT   CLOTHING SIZE   WAIST   INSEAM   OUTSEAM   SHOE SIZE

_____

_____

_____

Talents: Voice ___ Instruments ___ Dance ___ Languages ____ Acting Experience ____
••
DO NOT PRINT BELOW THIS LINE. FOR OFFICE USE ONLY: SAG___ AFTRA ___

Reg Date _____ Cntrct Date _____ Print ___ Film ___ Voice Over ___ SPCL ___

Pink: Girls   Yellow: Boys

PRINT LAST NAME	FIRST	INITIAL		#1 PHONE	#2 PHONE
ADDRESS		CITY		STATE	
SOCIAL SECURITY #		BIRTH DATE	TODAY'S DATE		ZIP CODE

MEN	SUIT SIZE	SHIRT	CHEST	WAIST	INSEAM
WOMEN	DRESS SIZE	BUST	WAIST		HIPS
CHILDREN	DRESS SIZE		SUIT SIZE		

EYES	HAIR	HOSE	HEIGHT S/F
HAT	GLOVE	SHOE	PHOTO RATE

UNIONS

FILM ☐	PHOTO ☐	FASHION ☐	VOICE ☐
CONVENTION ☐	HANDS ☐	LEGS ☐	☐

Dear Susan,

Thank you for giving us the opportunity to consider you for representation by our Agency,

I am sorry to say that we are not in a position to proceed any further at this time. We have numerous candidates requesting representation by our Agency. Consequently, competition among models is intense. As a result, we have identified candidates with overall qualifications which more closely meet the needs of our clients at this time.

Let me assure you that your candidacy received very careful review. We genuinely appreciate your interest,
                                        and wish you much success in your pursuit of a modeling career.

Sincerely,

President

REJECTION LETTER

23

Work Permits

Why does my child need a work permit? The answer is simple: for the protection and well-being of your child and the agency. Most agencies will require a work permit in the child's name, which protects the agency in case anything happens to your child on the job. (See sample work permits.) If an agency does not send you information about how to obtain a work permit, contact your state Department of Labor to find out what is required. I received from my first agency a "Letter of Intent" form, stating to the local schools or Department of Labor, whichever applies (where you go to obtain a work permit differs from state to state), that the agency intended to try to find jobs for my child in the modeling or acting field. In Illinois I had to visit our physician for an evaluation of my child, which stated that he was healthy and carried no communicable diseases; in Michigan this is required only up to a certain age. I also had to supply an official sealed copy (not a photocopy) of my son's birth certificate; and a letter giving my permission for my son to work in this field. After assembling these materials, I had to bring them, along with Jason, to a downtown Chicago office in order to receive his work permit. After that first year, I found out I could go to the high school in our area instead of to the city. In Michigan, contacting the Department of Labor is the route to follow.

Four of the five agencies my son was registered with required a work permit in the agency's name; one agency accepted a copy of one of the other agencies. Once you have a work permit issued for each agency which sent you a Letter of Intent, keep one copy and turn one copy in to the agency for its files. It is *my* responsibility to renew the work permits in the same manner each year and again send in the original copy to the agency. The work permit must be carried with us on all jobs and shown if requested. If you do not keep the work permits current, your child may not be called for auditions until the permit is renewed.

It is a good idea to study the rules and laws regarding the times your child can work. For instance, I encountered the following situation; When Jason was eight, he was called to appear in a commercial without an audition and was booked based on his composite and strong resume. The commercial would pay three-hundred dollars. However, there was a catch—the time of the shoot was from 11:30

LAB⬥R

APPLICATION FOR PERFORMING ARTS AUTHORIZATION
MICHIGAN DEPARTMENT OF LABOR/BUREAU OF SAFETY AND REGULATION
WAGE HOUR DIVISION
7150 HARRIS DRIVE, P. O. BOX 30015
LANSING, MI 48909
TELEPHONE: 517/322-1825

Act 90 Public Acts of 1978, as amended,
Deviation of hours cannot be granted unless this
form is completed and returned to the above address
for review and approval.

The Michigan Department of Labor will not discriminate
against any individual or group because of race, religion, age,
national origin, color, marital status, handicap or political
beliefs.

EMPLOYER INFORMATION

Steps to follow

1. Answer all questions. The processing will be delayed if you do not answer all the questions.
2. Print or type only.
3. Employer or authorized representative of employer must sign the application.
4. Application must be made for each production.
5. Written permission of the parent or guardian must be submitted with this application.
6. Attach doctor's statement verifying the performance will not be detrimental to the minor's health for minor under six years of age.

Important

1. If approved by the Department, the deviation is valid for the period indicated above.
2. Adult supervision must be present during the period the minor is working.
3. Authorization may be denied, suspended, or revoked by the Department when it is determined the employer is in violation with the provisions of Act 90.
4. When productions are performed that require the minor to be on tour during the school year, a state certified teacher must accompany the school age minor.

Name of Business:_____

Telephone: _____ Federal ID No. _____

Street Address:_____ County: _____

City: _____ State _____ Zip_____

Address where performance will take place if request is approved by the Department. (Attach listing if any additional locations where work is to be performed)

Street Address:_____ City:_____ County:_____

EMPLOYER STATEMENT

The above business requests approval to employ:

Name of Minor: _____ Birth Date:_____

Address: _____ Role to be performed: _____

Hours of Employment _____ Total hours per week _____

Dates of Performance: _____

Name of certified teacher accompany minor during school year: _____

REFER TO OTHER SIDE OF FORM FOR ADDITIONAL INFORMATION AND SIGNATURE

GUIDELINES FOR EMPLOYMENT OF MINORS BY PERFORMING ARTS ORGANIZATIONS

1. A minor should <u>not</u> be employed in establishments where alcoholic beverages are sold for consumption on the premises <u>unless</u> the sale of food or other goods constitutes at least 50% of the total gross receipts.

2. Infants who have reached the age of fifteen days but have not reached the age of six months may be permitted to remain at the place of employment for a maximum of two hours. The minor should not be employed between the hours of 9:00 p.m. and 6:00 a.m. The day's work should not exceed twenty minutes and under no conditions shall the infant be exposed to light of greater than one hundred foot candlelight intensity for more than thirty seconds at a time. A nurse must be provided for each ten or fewer infants.

3. Minors who have reached the age of six months but who have not attained the age of two years may be permitted at the place of employment for a maximum of four hours. Each four hour period should consist of not more than two hours of work. Minors aged six months to two years should not be employed between the hours of 9:00 p.m. and 6:00 a.m.

4. Minors between the ages of two years and five years may be permitted at the place of employment for a maximum of six hours. Each six hour period should consist of not more than three hours of work. Minors aged 2 years to five years should not be employed between the hours of 9:00 p.m. and 6:00 a.m.

5. Minors age six years to eight years may be permitted at the place of employment for a maximum of eight hours. Each eight hour period shall consist of not more than four hours of work. The minor shall not work between the hours of 10:30 p.m. and 6:00 a.m.

6. Minors age nine years to 13 years old may be permitted at the place of employment for a maximum of nine hours. Each nine hour period should consist of not more than 5 hours of work. On days when the minor's school is not in session the working hours may be increased to seven hours. Each minor should not work between the hours of 10:30 p.m. and 6:00 a.m.

7. A minor 14 years and over should not be employed between the hours of 11:30 p.m. and 6:00 a.m. when school is in session. The minor may be employed until 12:30 p.m. during summer school vacation periods or when the minor is not regularly enrolled in school.

8. Minors who have reached the age of fourteen years but who have not attained the age of eighteen years may be permitted at the place of employment for a maximum of ten hours on evenings preceding a day when the minor's school is in session; Each ten hour period shall consist of not more than six hours of work. On days when school is not in session, working hours may be increased to nine hours.

9. No minor shall be employed for more than 5 hours continuously without an interval of at least 30 minutes for a meal period. An interval of less than 30 minutes shall not be considered to interrupt a continuous period of work.

<u>Please advise the Department of the intent to deviate from any stated guideline.</u>

The Director of the Department of Labor may: Revoke this approval if the employment is determined to be detrimental to the health or personal well being of the minor, or if the minor is not adequately supervised or the minor's education is neglected.

NO PROVISIONS OF APPROVAL BY THE DEPARTMENT SHALL EXCUSE NONCOMPLIANCE WITH ANY OTHER FEDERAL OR STATE LAW OR MUNICIPAL ORDINANCE ESTABLISHING A MORE PROTECTIVE OR RESTRICTIVE STANDARD.

THE UNDERSIGNED CERTIFIES THE EMPLOYMENT WILL NOT BE DETRIMENTAL TO THE HEALTH, SAFETY, OR WELL BEING OF THE MINOR AND RECORDS WILL BE MAINTAINED AND MADE AVAILABLE FOR INSPECTION AT THE PREMISES WHERE THE MINOR IS EMPLOYED.

_____   _____
(Signature of employer or representative)   (Title)

_____   _____
(Print name of employer or representative)   (Date application signed)

STATE OF ILLINOIS
Department of Labor
Labor Law Enforcement Division
Thomas A. Graham, Supt.

Certificate No. _____

EMPLOYMENT CERTIFICATE

Date of Issue ____6-22-89____

VALID ONLY FOR MINOR AND EMPLOYER TO WHOM ORIGINALLY ISSUED

1. NAME OF SCHOOL __TINLEY PARK HIGH SCHOOL__ CITY __Tinley Park__ COUNTY __Cook__
2. This certifies that I, the undersigned issuing officer, have made a careful examination of all proofs, documentary or other wise, as required by Section 12 of the Act entitled "An Act to regulate the employment of children." approved June 30, 1945, in force and effect June 30, 1947 ___Jason Roy Randal Halter___ ___IL___ ___M___
   (Name of Minor)   (Address of Minor)   (Sex)
   and find the following: that this minor was born at __Evergreen Park__ __IL__
                                                        (City)   (State)
   ____Cook____ on the_____ day of __March__ , 19_____ ,
   (County)
   as shown by evidence of age __Certificate of Live Birth__ , and I have on file a statement from employer
                                (Name of Document Accepted)
   of intention to employ said minor; statement of physical fitness, and a statement of the principal of the school which the minor attends if this certificate covers employment during the school year
3. That the employer _____ _____ _____
                        (Name)   (Street)   (City)
   ____Model Agency____ , has promised the said minor present employment as a __Model__
         (Nature of Industry)   (Occupation)
   for __2__ on school days and not more than eight (8) hours on days when school is not in session, or _____
        (Hours)

   Is liquor served? Yes [ ] No [XX] — Summer Work only? Yes [ ] No [XX]

4. ____Susan M. Halter____ (Signature of Minor)   Susan M. Halter (Parent's Name and Address)
5. ____James Riordan____ (Superintendent of Schools)   Countersigned by ____Helen F. Jacob____ (Officer Authorized to Issues Employment Certificates)
6. ____TINLEY PARK HIGH SCHOOL____ (Name of School)   6111 W. 175th St. Tinley Park, IL 60477 (Address of School)

NOTE: Upon termination of employment of said minor, employer shall immediately return this certificate to the issuing officer.

ORIGINAL   SEE OTHER SIDE FOR CONDITIONS OF EMPLOYMENT
Send to Employer   Form No. LLE-25

STATE OF ILLINOIS AND FEDERAL CHILD LABOR LAWS
Employees subject to the State of Illinois and the Federal Labor Laws shall apply the higher standard
ILLINOIS CHILD LABOR LAWS

SECTION 3. HOURS OF WORK
"No minor under 16 years of age shall be employed, permitted, or suffered to work in any gainful occupation mentioned in Section 1 of this Act for more than 6 consecutive days in any one week, or more than 48 hours in any one week, or more than 8 hours in any one day, or be so employed, permitted or suffered to work between 7 P.M. and 7 A.M., except during the period June 1 to September 1, between 9 P.M. and 7 A.M. The hours of work of minors under the age of 16 years employed outside of school hours shall not exceed 3 a day on days when school is in session, nor shall the combined hours of work outside and in school exceed a total of 8 a day."

SECTION 4. MEAL PERIOD
"No minor under 16 years of age shall be employed, or permitted to work in any gainful occupation mentioned in Section 1 of this Act for more than 5 hours continuously without an interval of at least 30 minutes for meal period, and no period of less than 30 minutes shall be deemed to interrupt a continuous period of work."

SECTION 7. HAZARDOUS OCCUPATIONS (Excerpts)
"No minor under the age of 16 years of age shall be employed, permitted or suffered to work:
"In, about or in connection with any public messenger or delivery service, bowling alley, pool room, billiard room, skating rink, exhibition park or place of amusement, garage, filling station or service station, or as a bellboy in any hotel or rooming house or about or in connection with power-driven machinery.
"In any place or establishment in which intoxicating alcoholic liquors are served or sold for consumption on the premises, or in which such liquors are manufactured or bottled."
For further information contact Illinois Department of Labor, Labor Law Enforcement Division, 910 So. Michigan Ave, Chicago, Illinois, 60605, (312) 793-2804.

FEDERAL CHILD LABOR LAW
(As provided by the Fair Labor Standards Act — Section 3, 52 Stat. 1060, as amended; 29 U.S.C. 203).
14 and 15-YEAR-OLD MINORS MAY NOT BE EMPLOYED:
• During school hours, except as provided for under the Work Experience and Career Exploration Program.
• Before 7 A.M. or after 7 P.M. except 9 P.M. from June 1 through Labor Day (time depends on local standards).
• More than 3 hours a day — on school days.   • More than 8 hours a day — on nonschool days.
• More than 18 hours a week — in school weeks.   • More than 40 hours a week — in nonschool weeks.
14 and 15-YEAR-OLD MINORS MAY NOT BE EMPLOYED IN:
• Any Manufacturing occupation.
• Any Mining occupation.
• Processing occupations.
• Occupations requiring the performance of any duties in workrooms or workplaces where goods are manufactured, mined, or otherwise processed.
• Public messenger service.
• Operation or tending of hoisting apparatus or of any power-driven machinery.
• Any occupations found and declared to be hazardous.
• Occupations in connection with transportation, warehousing and storage, communications, public utilities, and construction.
Any of the following occupations in a retail, food service, or gasoline service establishment: Cooking (except at soda fountains, lunch counters, snack bars, or cafeteria serving counters) and baking; Occupations which involve operating, setting up, adjusting, cleaning, oiling, or repairing power-driven food slicers and grinders, food choppers and cutters, and bakery-type mixers; Work in freezers and meat coolers and all work in preparation of meats for sale (except wrapping, sealing, labeling, weighing, pricing and stocking when performed in other areas); Loading and unloading goods to and from trucks, railroad cars or conveyors.
The above is not all inclusive. For additional information, contact any office of the U.S. Department of Labor, Wage-Hour Division.

p.m. until 3:30 a.m., and on a school night! The child labor law at the time of this call stated that a child under the age of nine could not work between the hours of 10:30 p.m. and 6:00 a.m. But that is not the only reason why we did not accept the job. I am not so desperate to accept work for my boys that I would allow them to work at all hours of the night, and common sense told me to refuse it. So, you must ask yourself at times, where does one draw the line when accepting the shoot (job) for your child? Reinforcing the importance of looking out for our children's best interest should always be top priority.

See samples of work permits. However, these are only the current samples at the time this book went into print. They may vary from state to state, so make sure you obtain the most recent forms.

Multi-listed or Exclusive?

When Jason's career began, I waited and waited, thinking no talent agency was going to respond; however, we finally were contacted not by one agency but several. By registering with several agencies, Jason became multi-listed. Both of my boys are multi-listed, which at this time I prefer to exclusive listing,(which means being represented solely by one agency). I have heard a variety of conversations about exclusive listing. If you sign an exclusive contract (this is not the same as being registered; to register you do not sign a contract, you fill out, with most agencies, an information card) with one agency for, say, six months or one year, your child is the exclusive property of that agency. This means you cannot take any audition calls from any other agency or you will be in breach of contract with the agency with which you are exclusively listed. When your child is exclusively listed, you should be called more frequently by that agency than if your child were multi-listed.

I was under the impression in the beginning that going exclusive with one agency meant you had really made it. For a select few this could be true. But I have found out from others in the business that it does not always work out that way in practice. In fact, some parents could not wait until their exclusive contract expired. I think that by being multi-listed you are open to more opportunities.

28

Each talent agency receives different calls. Some do a lot of commercial work, at the national level or at the regional level; while others deal with casting agents who call for auditions for mini-series and films. Some strictly hire children who are not union members. Nevertheless, casting agents who notify the talent agents might not have your talent agency on their lists to notify for a particular audition. So by being multi-listed your chances are greater to be called more often.

A code of ethics exist for the multi-listed. At times, more than one agency has called to tell me about the same audition or has left a message on our home answering machine (a must-have). When that happens, I always write the name of the first agency to call me on the sign-in sheet at the audition, so that the agency which called me first will be the one to receive a commission, should my sons receive the job. If your child is exclusively listed, you would not have this problem, since only one agency would contact you for the audition.

Before we moved to Michigan, both of my boys were asked to be exclusively listed with one of our agencies in Chicago. It was a great offer, but we had to decline because remaining mult-listed offered more potential for us. It is your decision whether you have your child multi-listed or exclusively listed. If you decide to go exclusive, be sure to find out the specialties of your potential agencies before choosing one. Read the agency's contract from top to bottom; consulting an attorney is not a bad idea either. Know what you are signing.

CHAPTER 3

Pictures and Composites: How to Assemble an Inexpensive but Effective Portfolio

In this chapter, I will explain how I kept the agencies supplied with photos, the inexpensive way. As our children grow older we tend not to take as many photos of them as we did when they were babies: But remember, if your agency does not have photos, how can they promote your child? When I started out I was told by my first agency not to waste money on professional studio photographs. The cost could be close to two-or three-hundred dollars. Think about it: Your baby's appearance will change significantly every month until he or she is a year old, and every few months thereafter until about age four or five. After that, as children grow older, the changes are not so quick or dramatic. How often will you be willing to spend hundreds of dollars for new photographs?

Snapshots

Taking my own photographs still works well to this day with Jason (12) and Nicholas (10). All the agencies accept my photos and keep asking for more when they are out. From what I understand, most parents do resort to a professional photographer by the time their children are the ages of mine. My feeling is, why spend the money if it's not necessary? Having a good camera is an asset. Agencies like the pictures to be CLEAR and IN FOCUS, and showing only the child who is registered with the agency. Close-ups as well as full-length shots are important.

When I take pictures, I try to capture the personality of my boys. Taking pictures of children while they are active brings out their expressions. Jason has been booked for (received) many jobs as a result of his "action smiles," because, I have been told, it looks as if he were jumping right out of the picture. If you have a family member or a close friend who is a professional photographer and would be willing to help you out, that is great. I had the opportunity to do this once and received a contact sheet (see example), which allowed me to pick out the ones I wanted enlarged. A student photographer did the work without charge, just for the experience, and was happy to be part of the boys' career.

When I started in this business and my film was ready to be developed, I usually requested doubles. Then, I would pick my favorite poses and have numerous copies made. When I had a hard time getting a good close-up photo of my boys, I would go to the studio at my local department store and have close-up pictures taken there. Their prices were very reasonable and the quality of their work was good.

I have had my photographs developed throughout the years by mail-order photo labs. The mail-order film processor I use develops just about any brand of film, as well as its own. The prices for rolls of film and film processing are very low, and frequently the company runs special promotions on film. The drawback, of course, is the time delay. Mail-order processing takes longer then the same-day or next-day processing found locally. But, when I was not in a rush, I would send my film out for developing to save money.

Labeling Photographs

After taking the pictures myself, having them developed, choosing the best ones and ordering reprints, I was ready to send them to the agencies. But wait, first I had to write gently on the back of *each and every one* the following information; name, birthdate, age, social security number, height, weight, hair and eye color, size of clothing, date of the photo, and our address and telephone numbers, day and evening. Believe it or not, some parents even carry pagers and list those numbers as well, so they do not miss a single audition call for their child. If you

Contact Sheet

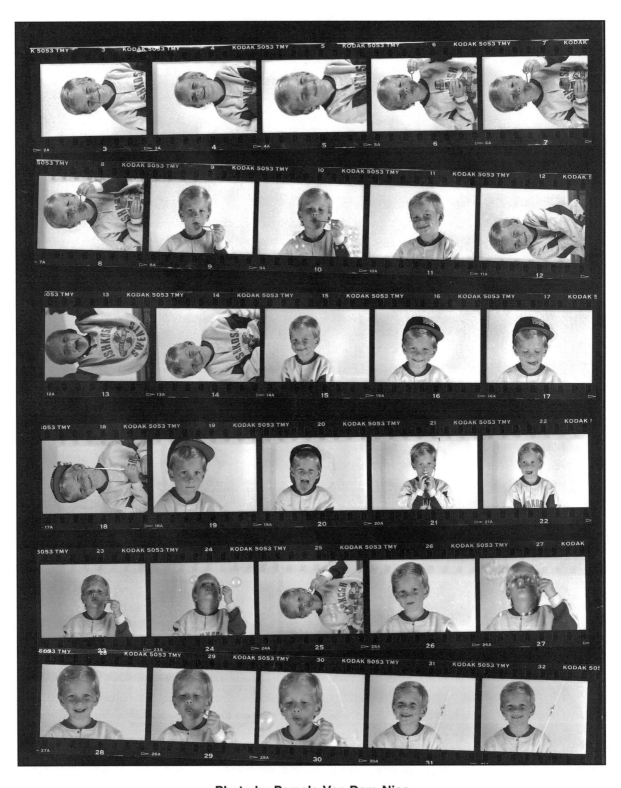

Photo by Pamela Van Dam-Njaa

Headsheet

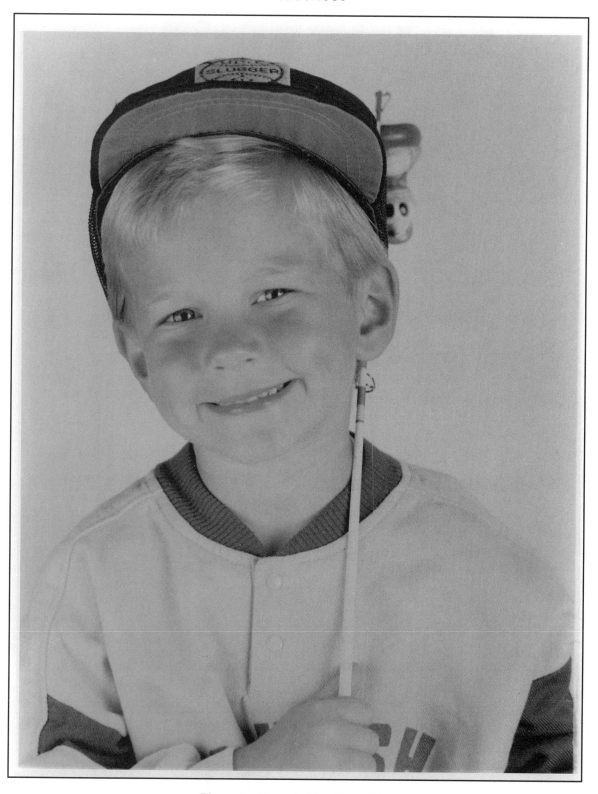

Photo by Pamela Van Dam-Njaa

Nicholas and Jason Halter Snapshots

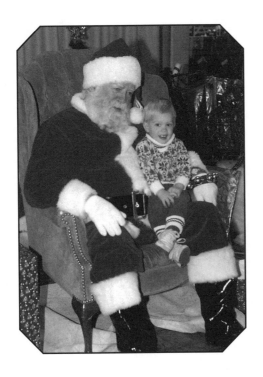

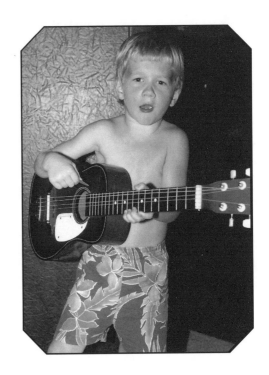

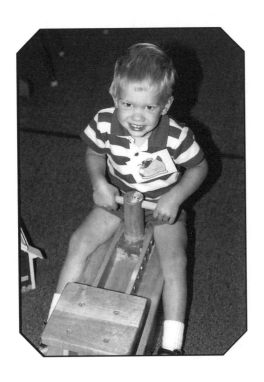

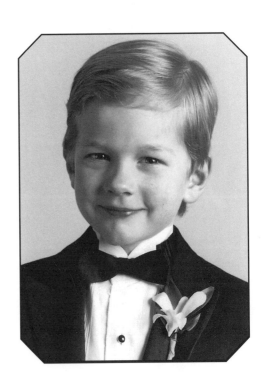

have a celluar phone, you might want to add that number to your information. I have been at auditions where mothers' pagers have gone off to tell them about another audition right after the one they were attending!

From the beginning, I also included on the back of photographs what activities my boys were doing, such as crawling, walking, riding a bike, and so on. Now I attach a resume. When I started, I supplied as much information as I could fit on the back of a photo. Doing so can only help the agency personnel know more about the person in the picture; they are not mind readers. Believe me, my hand would become cramped after completing about ten of those photographs, and remember, I was writing on almost fifty. If I were starting out now and had access to a computer, I would type the information I mentioned above, copy it, and adhere it to the back of each photo in a neat, clean way.

Composites

When Jason and then Nicholas turned four, it was time to think about putting a composite together instead of using loose snapshots (see sample composite). A composite is a group of photos, usually 8" x 10" in size printed on cardstock paper. Or many people use just a single photo, which is called a headshot, in 8" x 10" size also printed on cardstock. I favor using more than one photo and putting the statistics on the front or listing them on a separate sheet like a resume. As you can see, I used my imagination when putting the boys' resumes together. I began attaching the resumes to their composites, a resume being a listing of all the jobs one has done. Producers like to see if a child has worked before. Although a resume is not necessary, it helps to advertise the child's experience.

Usually, a composite is black and white. Color, which is more costly, is not necessary, although some people choose to have it. I do from time to time. One year, I changed to color composites for the agencies to see if it made a difference; however, it did not. We actually received more bookings when I was using the black and white. I have heard, though, that if your child has red hair it is a real plus to have a color photo. Agents like to see that red hair, and a black and white photo just does not do red hair justice. Again this is personal perference and the choice is yours.

After deciding which pictures to use and attaching them with a small piece of tape (on the back only, not the front) to a sheet of typing paper, I would send the composite layout in the mail to a company that specializes in processing composites, ABC Pictures (address listed under references, in back of book). When you send a photo layout through the mail, be sure to insert cardboard for support. The photographs, rather than negatives, are used to make a lithograph. The lithographed prints are on heavy 8-point floss-coated stock, and the company uses a fine 150-line-per-inch screen. The print resemble original "glossies" (a term used in the industry for an 8" x 10" headshot) so closely that the difference is seldom noticed. The price is unbelievable; I have to buy five hundred at a time, but who wouldn't when they cost only eighty-five dollars, or seventeen cents for each 8"x10" four-photo composite? I have not found a price like that anywhere else. Even though I usually do not use up the entire five-hundred, I have come pretty close, and for me it has been very cost effective.

Composite

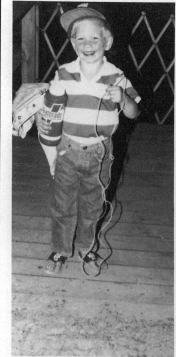

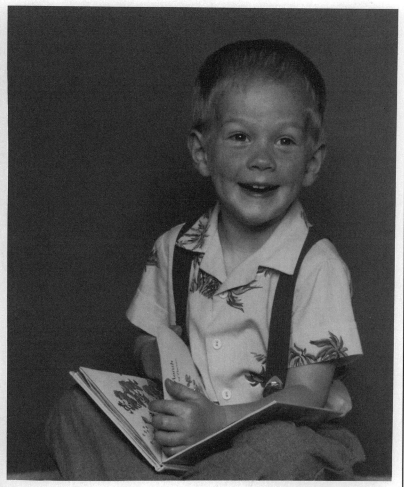

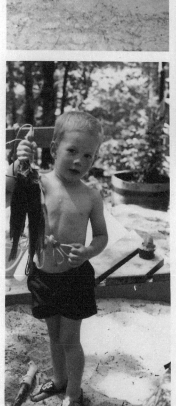

Jason Roy Randal Halter

HEIGHT	40"	BIRTHDATE	03-15-85
WEIGHT	32LBS.	WAIST	20"
HAIR	BLONDE	INSEAM	15"
EYES	BLUE	SHOE	9
SIZE	4-4T	S.S.#	

Resume

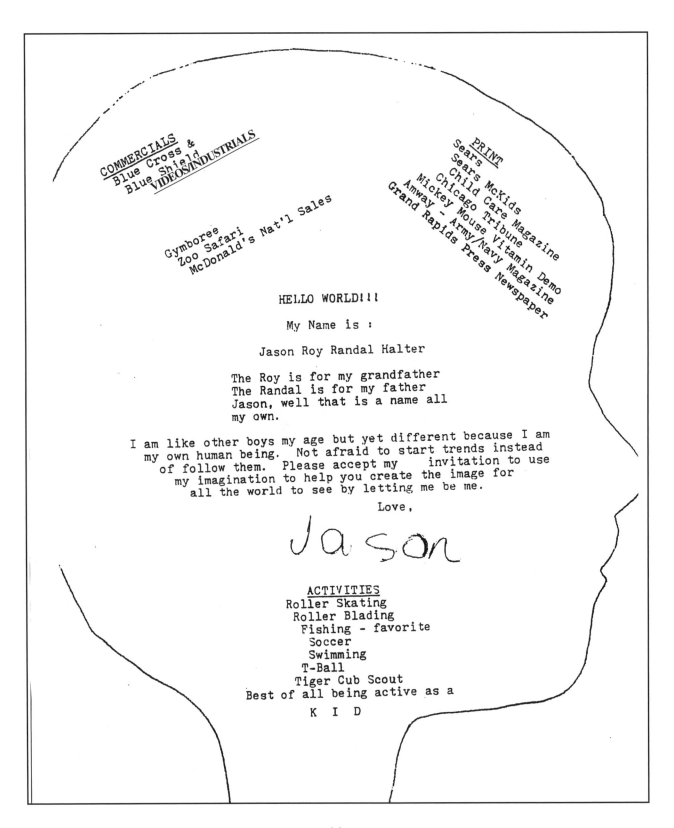

COMMERCIALS &
Blue Cross &
Blue Shield
VIDEOS/INDUSTRIALS

Gymboree
Zoo Safari
McDonald's Nat'l Sales

PRINT
Sears McKids
Sears
Child Care Magazine
Chicago Tribune
Mickey Mouse Vitamin Demo
Amway - Army/Navy Magazine
Grand Rapids Press Newspaper

HELLO WORLD!!!

My Name is :

Jason Roy Randal Halter

The Roy is for my grandfather
The Randal is for my father
Jason, well that is a name all
my own.

I am like other boys my age but yet different because I am
my own human being. Not afraid to start trends instead
of follow them. Please accept my   invitation to use
my imagination to help you create the image for
all the world to see by letting me be me.

Love,

Jason

ACTIVITIES
Roller Skating
Roller Blading
Fishing - favorite
Soccer
Swimming
T-Ball
Tiger Cub Scout
Best of all being active as a

K   I   D

Composite

Nicholas James Edward Halter

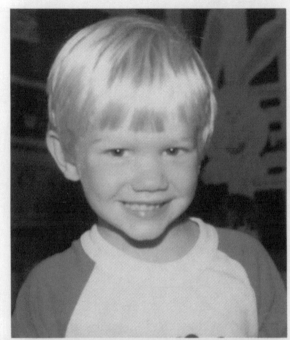

Height: 40"
Weight: 40 lbs.
Hair: Blonde
Eyes: Blue
Size: 4
Birthdate: 06-09-87
Waist: 21 1/2
Inseam: 15 1/2
Shoe: 10-11
S.S.#:

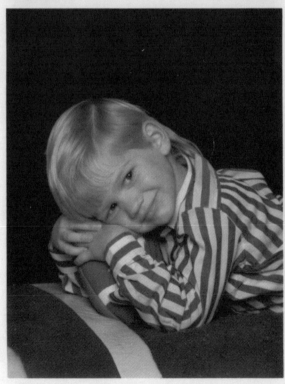

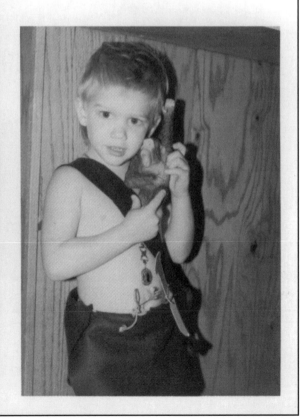

Resume

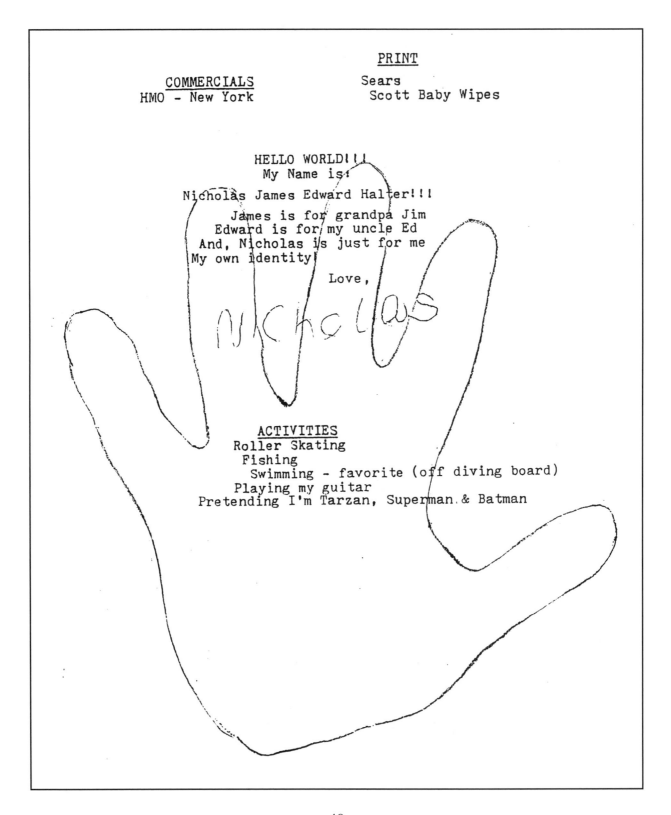

Laser Copy Machines for Fast Reprints

Since moving to Michigan, I have not been accepting as many audition calls from my boys' Chicago agencies because of the six-hour drive to and from Chicago plus a one-to-two-hour audition call. Therefore, I do not need nearly so many composites as I used to. It would be nice if attitudes changed within the industry and the Chicago casting agencies began accepting video auditioning for talent outside their market. It would make it easier for us to stay active in the Chicagoland area.

More recently, thanks to modern technology, I have been using a laser color photocopy machine to make composites from my own photographs of Jason and Nicholas. What prompted my experimentation with laser copy composites was a call from our Michigan agency informing me that it had no composites of Jason and wanted one ASAP to send to a casting director. (I should have been calling the agency every few months to make sure it had enough composites). Quickly, I called around to printing shops in my area to locate a laser-color copy machine. After finding one close by and arranging some current photographs of Jason, I had them copied at the shop and was pleased with the results. When I checked with the agency personnel regarding the possible continued use of the laser composites, the agency thought it would be just fine. However, I should warn you that not all laser copy machines have the same quality.

Because we don't need as many composites now as we used to, the laser copies are more cost effective for us. Nonetheless, if our situation changed and we needed a large number of composites at one time, I would go back to using ABC Pictures, Inc. Although I appreciate the convenience of being able to assemble a new composite with recently developed pictures at a moment's notice, making a hundred of them, at one dollar per copy, for example, would be too expensive. Being cost conscious, I look for the best deal for a given situation.

An Agency's Request for
Additional Materials

Guess What?

We are out of the following materials on you:

☐ Composites   ☐ Promotional Videos

☒ Headshots/~~Resumes~~   ☐ Voice Cassettes
there is still time to go on the 1994 headsheet. We need a
black/white, 8 by 10, headshot @ $75.00 ASAP.

Please Call

as soon as possible!

Jason Roy Randal Halter
Composite

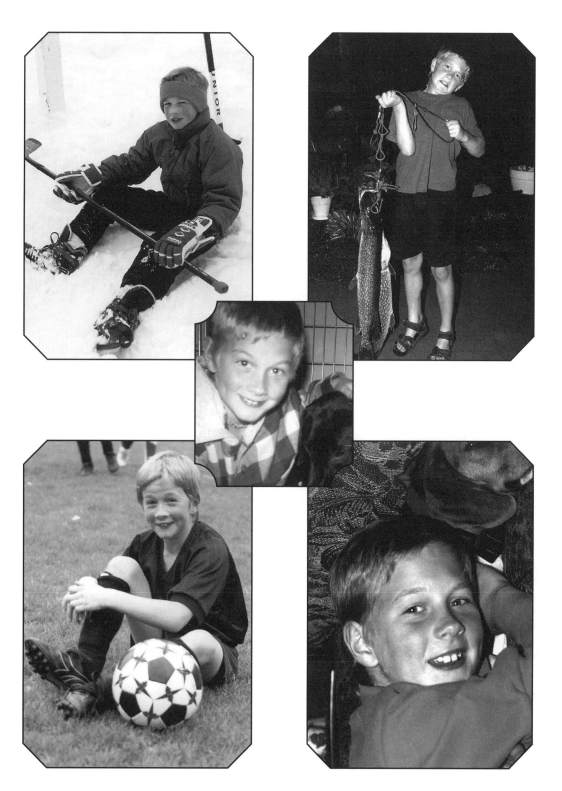

Resume

COMMERCIALS

Blue Cross & Blue Shield
Danne's Food Markets

VIDEO/INDUSTRIAL

Gymboree - GymVideo
Zoo Safari
Amway National Sales Videos
Whirlpool Appliances

PRINT

Blue Cross & Blue Shield
Sears
Sears McKids
Child Care Magazine
Mickey Mouse Vitamins
Amway
Grand Rapids Press
Fry Foundation - Cover

MISCL

Ava Anthony Productions

HELLO WORLD!!!

My Name is

JASON ROY RANDAL HALTER

The Roy is for my Grandfather
The Randal is for my Father
And Jason, well that is me
My own identity

I am a professional kid at heart. Please accept my invitation to use my imagination to help you create an image for all the world to see by letting me be me.

ACTIVITIES

Love Fishing
Ice Skating
Hockey
Snow skiing
Roller blading
Swimming - love the diving board
Soccer

Shooting my bow & arrow
Bike riding
Skating Boarding
Snowmobiling
Cub Scouts - 5th year
And best of all just being a kid

STATISTICS

Height: 57"
Weight: 77lbs.
Hair: Blonde
Eyes: Blue
Size: 10
Birthdate:
Waist: 25"
Inseam: 21"
Shoe: 3/4
SS#
Agencies: Chicago, IL and
Grand Rapids, MI
Experience from 6 wks old
Date of composite 9/94

Nicholas James Edward Halter
Composite

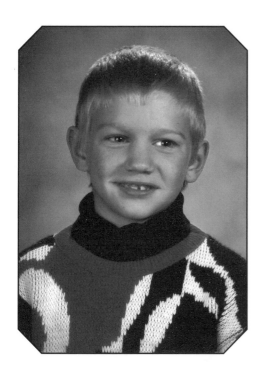

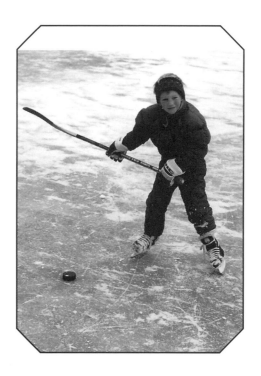

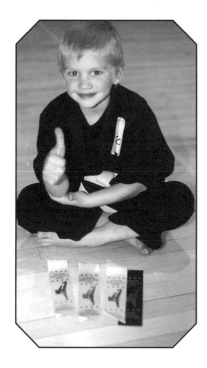

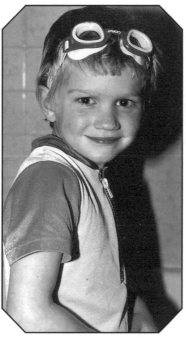

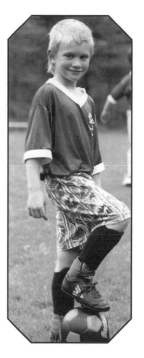

Resume

COMMERCIALS

HMO - New York

PlayWorld

PRINT

Scott Baby Wipes
Sears

HELLO WORLD

My Name is

Nicholas James Edward Halter

James is for Grandpa Jim
Edward is for Uncle Ed
And Nicholas is just for me
My own identity

ACTIVITIES

Roller Blading
Ice Skating
Hockey
Speed Skating
Karate - Green belt
Swimming
Soccer
Snow Skiing
Bike riding
Cub Scout 2nd year
And just being a kid

STATISTICS

Height: 45"
Weight: 50lbs.
Hair: Blonde
Eyes: Blue
Size: 7
Birthdate:
Waist: 20 1/2"
Inseam:16"
Shoe: 13
SS#
Agencies: Chicago, ILand
Grand Rapids, MI
Experience from 6 wks old
Date of composite 9/94

Agency Kids' Book or Kids' Poster

What is a Kids' Book or Kids' Poster? A talent agency could at some point, after you have registered with them (free of up-front charges), invite your child to appear in either the agency's poster of headshots of the kids who are registered with them or in the agency's Kids' Book or Talent Book. Agencies all have their own name for it. These books or posters are usually kept in the agency offices or sent to casting agents to look at if requested. When you visit a talent agency, you will see on the walls posters of children represented by that agency. I have heard that some casting people don't bother looking at these books or posters because they think that the children pictured have probably changed since the printing, which is probably true for certain age groups. On the other hand, their are some casting agents that appreciate having the kids grouped together this way.

Appearing in the promotional book or poster is not free. Some agencies let you send in your own photos, but they will specify the size, type of shot, etc., and some will want you to go to a specific photographer, to make the shot super clear. One agency wanted us to go to its photographer only and would not accept pictures from us. I was a little leery about this. Remember, this is what we are supposed to watch out for. But, like so many things, there are exceptions to the rule. After asking many questions and seeing what I would receive for my money, I realized that the photographer was not making a great profit, and the agency request was legitimate and based on a concern that the photo be of professional quality for this particular situation. Jason has appeared in both the poster and the book. Nicholas appeared in just the poster. It did not seem to make much difference in the number of auditions they received whether they were included in the poster or the book or neither. Following is a picture of Jason that appeared in an agency book.

PHOTOGRAPH TAKEN FOR
AGENCY CHILDRENS' BOOK

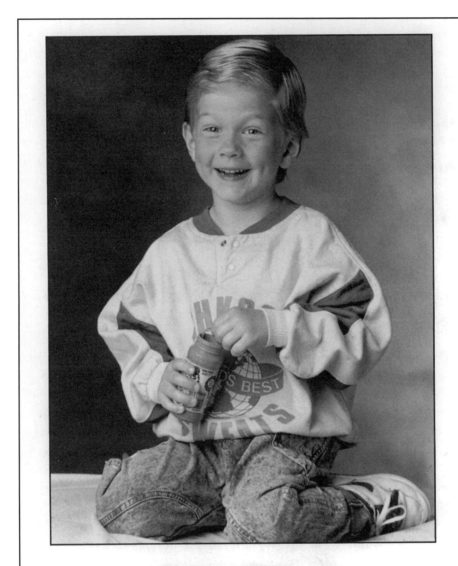

Jason Halter

Size: 4-5   Height: 40"   Weight: 38
Waist: 19   Inseam: 15   Outseam: 21
Hair: Blonde   Eyes: Blue   Shoe: 9   S.S.
Birthdate: 3-15-85

Photo by Richard Dionisio

CHAPTER 4

The First Audition: How to Prepare and What to Expect

*O**ur first audition!*** Well, if you can call it that. The unusual often happens to us. After sending the photographs, work permits and registration cards to the agencies, I had to wait only a couple of weeks before I received our first call (the day before Jason's first birthday) for not only an audition but also a regional union commercial booking for a very well known healthcare insurance company. The call was based solely on Jason's snapshots. What a way to start! Although I now know that commercials are few and far between, at the time I thought, "What a piece of cake! Who said this business is full of rejections? Jason is one-for-one and didn't even have to audition. Plus, it is a commercial with residuals!" The fee paid for each broadcast of a commercial after the initial airing. The amount varies depending how many times, over what length of time and in what markets the commercial is shown. Also the size of the performer's roll is a factor to determine the residual rate. Well, let's say it was beginner's luck, being the right age or having the right look or being available when the baby who was called before Jason, could not do the job. Call it whatever, but remember that although you can speculate, you usually don't really know why a certain person does or does not get a particular job.

Landing a job without an interview was a rare accomplishment; real auditioning soon followed. Although we have gone to numerous auditions since then, my boys have not had another lucrative commercial job like that one which paid residuals. Whenever my boys do not receive a job from an audition or are not requested at a call back (a request for a second audition, which is not unusual but does not always occur), I mark it up as experience and still feel good that they were at least halfway there because they had been chosen for the audition from among thousands of registered children. I stopped trying to figure out why they sometimes do not get a commercial and learned not to take the rejection personally. "It is not worth worrying about. Just let it go," I always tell myself.

Real auditioning starts with a phone call from one of our talent agencies. I keep a pen or pencil and paper near my telephone so that when I am called by a talent agent regarding an audition, I will be able to record important information such as time, place, required attire, and so on. (Talent agents are busy; do not make them wait while you search for a pencil or paper.) A carbonless phone message book in duplicate makes a great message pad. I use one, so I always have a second copy of my notes in case I have to refer back at a later time. A pad of this sort can be purchased at most office supply stores. I also keep at hand a list of my boys' current statistics, in case the agent requests them. If one of my boys has a recent cut or scab or a bruise from a fall, and it would show in pictures or on film, I do not accept an audition invitation without first telling the agent about the disfigurement and letting him or her decide whether we should come. Sometimes it matters and sometimes it doesn't.

At times you have only a few hours' notice when you are called for an audition. Usually you have a scheduled audition time; otherwise the audition is considered a "cattle call," where you can arrive at any time between certain hours; but so can everyone else the agency has contacted, as well as all the other talent from the various agencies that were called by the casting people too. I prefer the scheduled-time auditions, which are much more organized most of the time.

As a result of an audition call, my whole day, from that call on might be rearranged and refocused on preparing for the audition. I start by making sure everyone is clean and neat (if not, into the shower or tub they go); laying out appropriate clothes (ironing them if necessary); and checking to see that their shoes are presentable.

Preparing for the Audition

All right, are we ready to go to the audition? Wait! Not so fast. Did I ask all the necessary questions? For example; Will there be call backs? If so, when? When will the actual take place? Is this a union or non-union job and if it is union which union? If I have other shoots or callbacks or other time conflicts on the shoot date, I have to tell the agency. On some rare occasions, if a casting director or producer who already knew Jason and Nicholas wanted either of them enough, he worked around our schedule. I would just always make sure first, because there is no sense in going to an audition if you know you cannot make the callback or the shoot date.

Next question; Do I know where I am going? Don't laugh, we have had to wait over two hours past scheduled call times, for the other talent to show up because they were driving around in circles trying to find the address. Even if the agency gives me directions, I have learned to indicate the route on a street map before I leave my home for both the audition and the actual booking because if I have been given wrong directions, it is better to find out before I leave home when it's easier to call for the right directions. I learned that lesson the hard way when I was enroute with Nicholas for a commercial shoot. We were over a hundred miles away from home and had been given the wrong information about where to exit the highway. I rode more than half an hour out of my way, looking for the right street before stopping at a police station; (the safest place to stop when in unfamiliar places); to call the agency that had booked the job. I found out that everyone had been given the wrong directions and most were late and probably doing the same thing I was, panicking. If you can afford a celluar phone, I recommend that you have one. If I had had a car phone, I could have called the agency from my car. So you see why mapping out your route is so important before you leave. Because trying to read a big map while driving is not safe, I like to draw the route on a smaller piece of paper which I can safely consult. In addition, drawing the map helps me form a mental image of where I am supposed to go. When I am too far from home and my street map does not cover that area, I now stop and pick up a the local street map as soon as I enter the area. If I had done so for this particular job, after looking at the map, I would have realized I was not going to find the street by going in the direction I was headed.

Allowing extra time to drive to the audition or actual job is a sensible practice, not only for the reason above, you never know what you might run into; heavy traffic, especially during rush hours; accidents; road construction; bad weather, and so on. In cold climates, winter traveling can really test your nerves. I allow at least an extra hour when I have to drive from my home in Michigan to Chicago. But when the audition or job is close to home, I add only fifteen minutes to half hour to the expected driving time.

Although things do happen that are beyond our control, it is important to arrive on time for an audition or job. Being late for an audition or a shoot is a bad practice, because, if producers or directors have to wait for the talent, they probably won't forget it. I can only imagine what costs are incurred for a union commercial. In Chicago, I have noticed there are many more people on the sets than in Michigan. Although not so many people are involved in smaller productions, time is money in any market.

Sometimes, however, no one can predict or prevent a delay. Jason was once called to appear in a McDonald's birthday national sales video (known as an industrial video). After we arrived on the set, we overheard conversations about the two main characters; They were late, very late, and they had an earlier filming time than we did. Most producers will not have all the talent arrive at the same time, only as they are needed. As it turned out, on another highway, different from the one we had taken, a tanker had turned over, causing the highway to be closed. There was nothing anyone could do but rearrange the day's shooting schedule, and include the main characters when they arrived. Fortunately, everything worked out well in the end.

What to Bring

Let's see, I think I am ready to leave now. I have clean boys who are nicely dressed and my route is mapped out. . . .   But wait, my boys, like most children, become thirsty and hungry and want to keep busy while riding in the car and waiting at the audition. When Jason and Nicholas were very young keeping them content was much more difficult than it is now. I always brought plenty of entertainment items, especially if I thought we would have to wait long, as we did at "cattle calls." From time to time, I was known at the auditions as the "mom who keeps the kids occupied," not only my own but the others as well. I read books to them, started games and led songs. The other children in the room would hear what we were doing and come over and sit down and join us. Although I did these things to keep my boys from becoming bored while waiting for their audition time, I had fun too. If you don't keep younger children occupied while waiting, they might become irritable before the audition.

I also bring water and snacks, anything that does not stain clothes, of course. And, speaking of clothes, bring an extra set in case something happens to the ones they are wearing on the way. And, in our case, it has! Several times, Jason has fallen while getting out of the car, once tearing a hole in the knee of his pants. One hot summer day when Nicholas had just begun to walk, I did not put his socks and shoes on him before we left; instead, I just grabbed them from the shelf and put them in a bag. Later, I was alarmed to discover that I had taken two left shoes; one was Nicholas' and one was Jason's. They were the same shoe style but obviously not a pair. Luckily, I had an extra pair included with the back-up clothes I had prepared earlier.

Even though the boys are older now, we still have funny mishaps occasionally. When Jason was nine, he received a present of some entertaining slimy stuff, which is not supposed to stick to anything. He brought it on a trip to an audition and decided to put it around his neck. He said, "Look, Mom, a necklace!" Yes, it stuck to his shirt and some of it would not come off. Still, after all these years, I bring extra clothes. It buys peace of mind. Now that they are older, each boy packs his own goodie box with what he wants to entertain himself. Sometimes we have to wait anywhere from ten minutes to a hour, even though we have a scheduled audition time; so I always try to come prepared for a wait.

We still haven't finished packing our audition bag - - photographs! Usually the people running the audition take a instant picture, but they also want one of our photos as well as a resume if available. We are not always reminded by the talent agency to bring photos or a composite, so I have to remember to bring them.

Finally, We've Made it to the Audition

Yes, we have arrived at the audition! Many people have asked me what it's like at an audition. For children, as you know, waiting can be very difficult. At most of the auditions my boys and I have been to, we have had to sit in a small, sometimes very small, waiting room with about thirty people crowded together, at least half of them children, which has led to some uncomfortable situations. One time, a little girl was running up and down the hall outside the waiting room area while her mother was talking and not paying attention to her whereabouts. Moms love to talk about what their kids have done and how many auditions they have to go to that day. I'd rather not; that is why I choose to entertain the kids instead. Anyway, before long, the little girl walked right into the room where an audition was taking place. Needless to say, the people running the audition were upset by the intrusion. By keeping children busy and happily entertained, parents help everyone concerned.

When we enter the audition waiting room, I have to sign in on a couple of different sheets. Each producer or casting agent seems to have his or her own, but the information they usually request is the child's name, social security number, gender, and ethnicity; the parent's address and phone numbers; and the name of the agency that sent you (you must remember which agency called you first if you are multi-listed). The last item is important so that the people in charge will know which agency to contact if they want you for a call back or, if no call backs, for the actual job. Then someone from the talent agency calls you with the information the agency has received from the casting agent or director regarding the final details. On rare occasions, you may be contacted by the casting agent as well as the talent agent, especially if the audition is one day and the actual job is the next. Most talent agents go home like everyone else at the end of the day. So, occasionally, the casting people will call the talent, to let them know the details for the next day. Usually, however, the talent agency personnel do all the calling.

There is also a casting information sheet (see sample) which asks for the child's size, height, weight, and so on; whether your have any conflicts with the product, or other dates booked on their callback dates or shoot dates; and whether your child is a union member. After filling out these sheets, sometimes I have to

AUDITION SHEET
SIGN IN

NAME	ADDRESS	PHONE #	SS#	AGENCY	ACTUAL CALL TIME	IN	OUT	AGE+40	AGE-40	M /F

write each of my boys' names on a sheet of paper in large letters or on a clapboard, so that when the boys go into the audition, they can hold up the paper and identify themselves in front of the camera.

Next, we might be given instructions regarding lines to learn, if appropriate. Or we might receive the story lines, which are just like a mini-script (see my own example). I go over the story lines with Jason or Nicholas to familiarize them with the commercial they will be auditioning for. After we moved to Michigan, some of the Chicago agencies began giving us, a little more advance notice regarding an audition; and when there was a script involved for speaking parts in a movie or commercial, they would fax it to me so the boys could start practicing their lines. When the boys do not have to deliver lines during an audition, I sometimes have to drag out of them what they were asked when they went in. Being a curious parent, I am interested in their experiences. You know how talkative some kids can be. I usually ask, "How did it go? What did they ask you to do?" Many times, their reply is, "Oh, nothing" or "The usual," which means, they were asked their name, what they like to do, or whether they like being here and auditioning.

Once the paperwork is completed and the lines practiced, we just wait for Jason or Nicholas to be called for their time to shine! This might surprise you, but at the auditions we have attended in Chicago, parents are not allowed to go into the audition room with their children, even if the children are babies. The person running the audition takes the child, and the parent waits. In contrast, this is not so in West Michigan; parents are welcome to watch their child's audition. Having had the opportunity to do both, I prefer not to go in and only do so if either of the boys really wants me to. Although I enjoy seeing what goes on and how my boys do, I think their attention is much more focused on what they are doing when I am not in the room. If only audition sites had two-way mirrors for parents to view!

I'll never forget one of the first auditions I attended when Jason was a baby. When Jason's name was called, I stood up with him in my arms, and was walking towards the audition room when the assistant told me that she would take him from there. Being surprised and feeling anxious, I asked to see the room where he would have his audition. I looked around the room to see if there were any other exits. Being a new parent and entering a new territory, I wasn't going to take any chances of letting my child go in a room with strangers that I did not feel safe about. As

Casting Information Sheet
(Example sheet only)

DATE <u>January 5, 1997</u>

Advertising Agency   <u>Halter Advertising (example only)</u>

Client/Product<u>   Rancho Fries   </u>

Product Conflicts are<u> Example - Halter Fries   </u>

Shoot Date(s)<u>   January 15, 1997   </u>

Callbacks schedule<u>   January 10, 1997   </u>

****

(Please Print)

Name:_____S.S.

#_____

Age:_____ Birthdate:_____

Parent's Name(s) (if under 18

yrs):_____

Address:_____

           (Street)   (City/State)

Telephone #(s):_____

Agent (if you have

one):_____

Member of SAG (please circle one):   YES   NO   Taft-Hartley

****

Circle one of the following: Girl   Boy   Man   Woman

Height_____   Weight_____   Shirt_____   Slack_____

Dress_____   Jacket_____   Waist_____

Inseam_____

Shoe_____   Hat_____

****

Commercials/roles you have been a part of:

_____

_____

_____

Signature_____

Parent's Signature (if under 18 yr. old)who is the same height, skin tone, and hair

Story Board

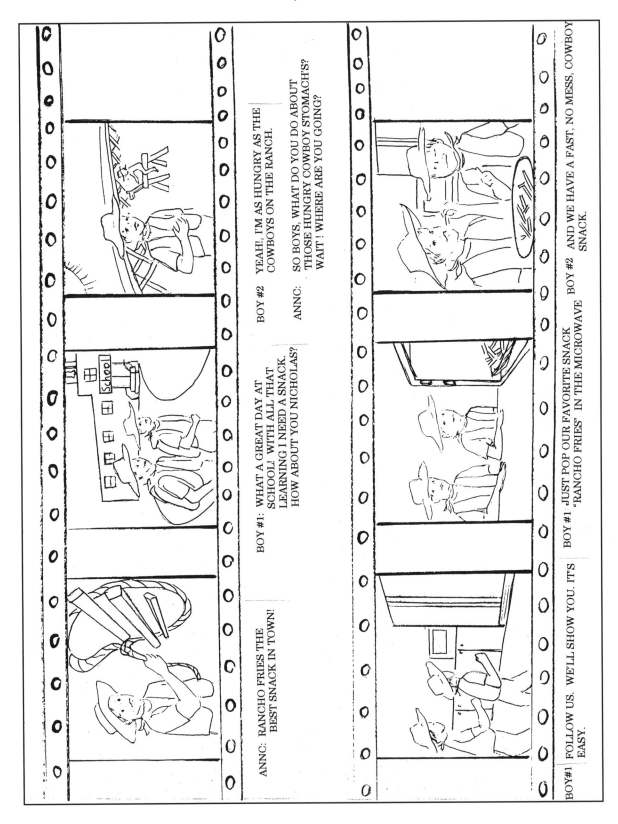

ANNC: RANCHO FRIES THE
BEST SNACK IN TOWN!

BOY #1: WHAT A GREAT DAY AT
SCHOOL! WITH ALL THAT
LEARNING I NEED A SNACK.
HOW ABOUT YOU NICHOLAS?

BOY #2 YEAH!, I'M AS HUNGRY AS THE
COWBOYS ON THE RANCH.

ANNC: SO BOYS, WHAT DO YOU DO ABOUT
THOSE HUNGRY COWBOY STOMACHS?
WAIT ! WHERE ARE YOU GOING?

BOY#1 FOLLOW US. WE'LL SHOW YOU. IT'S
EASY.

BOY #1 JUST POP OUR FAVORITE SNACK
"RANCHO FRIES" IN THE MICROWAVE

BOY #2   AND WE HAVE A FAST, NO MESS, COWBOY
SNACK.

time passed and I returned to the same places, I felt more comfortable releasing Jason for the auditions.

When your child is a baby, the separation test will help you decide whether your child should be in this business at that time. If he or she will not separate from you or will not cooperate during the audition, you will probably lose the job. The directors and producers need kids who can temporarily separate from their parents, which only makes sense. Can you blame them? Sure, kids will have good and bad days; that is normal, but if the bad days continue, read the signs and act accordingly. This experience should be fun for both of you. I like to give my boys a thumbs up sign and a hug when they go into an audition and a big hug when they return. I am trying to help them build their self-esteem and self-confidence just for being themselves.

I am glad I started my boys in print and commercial work when they were young. Now that they are old enough to know what they are doing, it is just a part of their life, another activity they do, like baseball, soccer, Cub Scouts, and Jason's love for fishing. I realized this when Jason went to an audition in Michigan and the producer of the commercial asked Jason if he liked doing "this type of stuff." Jason threw his hand out and said nonchalantly, "Oh, I do this all the time in Chicago." That remark helped Jason get the commercial for Daane's Food Market in Grand Rapids. The producer told me he liked the fact that Jason enjoyed what he was doing, that he was a natural and comfortable with it, and that Mom was not telling him he had to do it. Your child will tell the truth about whether he or she wants to be in this business. I heard a casting director tell a group of people that when she interviews a child, the first question she asks is, "Do you want to be here?" or "Do you like being here?" If the answer is "No" the audition is over. Unfortunately, she does not have time to explain the rejection to each and every parent of a child who responds in that manner. So it is important to read the signs when children are very young and talk to them about their work as they grow older. It makes no sense to waste so many people's time if the child does not like auditioning.

The Waiting Game...

Whew! We made it through the audition and returned home. When we started in this business, going home after an audition was terrible. I usually knew what the dates for the callbacks and shoots were, so until they passed, I was a nervous wreck. Every time the phone rang, I jumped up, thinking, "Maybe this is the call." A telephone answering machine comes in handy in this line of work. As I look back, I see that I was definitely acting like a "new mom in the field." I couldn't sleep at night, wondering if my son would be given the job. The days passed and I would be sad, trying like crazy to figure out what went wrong. Only later did I learn to relax. It wasn't anything Jason or Nicholas had done or not done.

Who Is Chosen?

Many factors are involved in deciding which child is chosen for a job. Usually the decision is made by a group of people; the advertising staff, the client, the casting director, and the producer. They are searching for a certain look for a particular ad. Several times, my boys have been grouped with actor moms and dads or brothers and sisters, whom they have to resemble. The people in charge are trying to put many factors together to see what works best for the shot they want. If my boys have the look they want, great; if not, they at least have one more auditioning experience. I have learned not to take it personally.

No matter how excited I might be, I used to be careful not to talk about auditions in front of my sons and would distract them if the topic came up in conversations they could hear. There are people who do not see this business as I do, and their reactions to some situations are not what I care to have my boys listen to. Adjustments have to be made at each age level. For example, now that the boys are older, if their work comes up in conversation, we talk more openly and sometimes joke about it; "Oh well, I guess they picked the red-headed boy for that one; he did seem to fit in better with the red-haired actor dad." We even watch for the commercials they have auditioned for and find out who did get the part. It's fun!

Keeping Records of Auditions

After the first year, I started keeping track of all the auditions we went to by writing them in a notebook. I have found it helpful to keep the names and addresses of and directions to the places we have gone to for auditions, especially since we do go back to some places again. Having those notes saves time for me and the agency staffs, who do not have to give me the same directions again. If you can be one step ahead of them they really appreciate it. The notes also tell me what kind of a year the boys have had. This is truly an up and down business. One year, the auditions might result in several jobs and the following year, just two. Then the total is up again the next year. I have heard from other parents that this variation is not unusual. For the average child, work comes in spurts. Just stick with it and make sure your agency always has up-to-date pictures on file otherwise, the agency staff cannot promote your child.

When I call in every once in a while to make sure they have enough photos on hand then, while I am on the phone, I can ask if there is anything going on for kids. Often, in the beginning, they would not remember my childrens names, but if I happened to call on a day when they had a audition scheduled for their age, we would be sent to the audition. I realized that the agency registered thousands of children. How would they get to know my boys unless I kept checking with them? However, you have to be careful not be become a pest. Use common sense while trying to make your child familiar to the agency staff.

Stand In's

Don't be surprised if your child doesn't get an actual job from an audition but is called back by the producer as a "stand in," at an agreed-upon rate. Jason was up for a national Sun-Maid Raisin commercial. I was told he was a favorite, but the job went to another boy. Why? When Jason found out he actually had to eat the raisins, he explained truthfully, "I don't care for raisins. No thank you for eating them." The producer appreciated his honesty and still used him as a "stand in" the day before the commercial was actually shot. A stand in is just that, a person who is the same height, skin tone, and hair color etc. as the person who will be featured in a commercial. Jason was hired just to sit in the same spots that were going to be shot, so lighting and position would be ready and no time, and therefore money, would be wasted when all the people were on the set.

Aspects of the Industry:
Fashion Shows, Printwork, Billboards, Product Packaging and Point of Purchase

Before my sons started working in this field, I did not realize it was divided into so many categories. It seems you don't learn about these different areas unless you are directly involved. I have searched for information about other aspects of the industry, even though my sons are not directly involved in them, because I want this book to be as useful as possible to people who are thinking about entering this business. Following are descriptions of other kinds of work your child may audition for:

FASHION SHOWS We have accepted only one fashion show job. The show was presented by a popular parents' magazine and was on tour for the back-to-school season. The models wore-name-brand clothes that you could purchase from stores in the Chicagoland mall where the fashion show was being held. I have not accepted work for my boys in fashion shows since then, because Jason, who was five at the time, was bothered to see everyone, male and female, dressing and undressing in the same room. I realize that this is what the backstage of a fashion show typically looks like, but it was not the right situation for Jason at the time. The scene backstage is very rushed and chaotic as the staff try to get all the models out and onto the runway when it is there cue. The pay is fair and determined by the number of shows in which the model participates. Often you are paid for your rehearsal time as well. A typical fashion show runs twice a day, one in the morning and in the afternoon, and could last thirty to forty-five minutes.

PRINTWORK This field can range from catalogs, newspapers and magazine covers to billboards. There is not a set rate for print and it varies quite a bit. Print work is usually paid by the hour. My sons' current rate in Michigan is from sixty-five to one-hundred dollars per hour, and in Chicago from seventy-five to one-hundred twenty-five per hour. They receive this rate because they are experienced; newcomers to the field probably will not start at this rate. If Jason or Nicholas is chosen at the hourly rate for a print job, he is paid the first hour's wage whether he works the full hour or not. Then he is paid in fifteen-minute increments. Print jobs can also be paid by the day or by the job. The agency's percentage is fifteen-to-twenty percent, depending on, for us, if the job is in Michigan or Chicago.

BILLBOARDS Have you walked through an airport lately? Or perhaps driven down the highway? Large or small billboards are everywhere and just another place an advertisement can appear. Billboard rates are usually paid by the day plus a bonus, depending on where the billboard ad will actually be placed, nationally or regionally.

PRODUCT PACKAGING If you look at a box of cereal in your cupboard it might have on it a picture of anyone from a famous basketball player, to an unknown little blonde-haired, blue-eyed boy. Well, that print work is known as "sight packaging" or "product packaging." It appears directly on the product you are buying. The pay is usually a day rate, plus bonuses.

POINT-OF-PURCHASE You see a large photograph on top of a pop display in a store with two boys, each holding a can of pop. This photo is at the point where the purchase is made, but not actually on the product. The rate, again is usually a day rate, plus bonuses. Again, depending on the product and the exposure.

Jason and Nicholas have not appeared in a point-of-purchase, product packaging, or billboard ads, but I have heard that some kids have earned up to fifteen-hundred dollars for just two hours of this type of work. Price negotiations for all of the above is done by the talent agent and usually the advertising companies calling for the talent. Again, these figures could vary greatly on all types of work other than union work.

Fashion Show For A
Popular Parents' Magazine

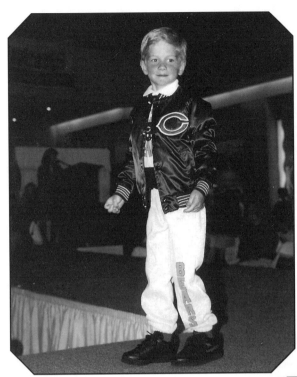

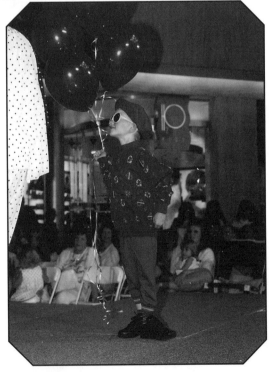

CHAPTER 5

The Day of the Job: What Goes Along with It and What Follows

Although highly unusual, our first call from an agency led to our first job—without an audition. Jason has permanently sketched his one-year-old smile in the commercial file for a major healthcare company in Iowa. At first, he was hired as an extra. The producer needed many crawling babies, and Jason, at the time, was still crawling but starting to take a few steps. If the call had come two weeks later, he probably would not have been given the job. (How do you keep a new walker down?) After receiving the call that Jason had been chosen, I was told to wait for my instructions from the people who were handling wardrobe. In Chicago, most of the jobs we have been booked for have had wardrobe persons, hair stylists, etc.; in Michigan, I usually do everything myself. What a difference living near a big city makes! Now that my boys are older, I am sometimes also sent a packet in the mail regarding a script if there is one, or just general information (see "Tips for Actors and Actresses Working in McDonald's Video Programs").

The next day I received a call from the person in charge of wardrobe, who told me to bring several of my son's outfits and shoes, and said that the producer would choose what Jason should wear. Those all-important directions were given regarding how to get to the shoot and what time to arrive. Because I allowed for extra travel time, which is always my practice, we arrived half an hour early that day and asked for the person in charge, who is usually the producer. I introduced

<u>Tips for Actors and Actresses</u>
<u>Working in McDonald's Video Programs</u>

Welcome to McDonald's Television Department.
Listed below are guidelines that will help you understand what we expect from you and what you will need to do in order to "look the part" for a McDonald's video program.

<u>CUSTOMERS:</u>

Please bring two complete non-seasonal outfits with you to the shoot. These outfits can be casual or work clothes (business suits to blue collar). Light sweaters and jackets are fine but, please, no shorts or heavy coats.

<u>CREW:</u>

Women - You must be able to put your hair up under the McDonald's caps so bring bobbie pins, hair clips, hair spray and whatever else you need to be able to accomplish this.

  - If you want to wear earrings, small stud earrings are the only acceptable earrings.

  - Your nails must be clean, short and neatly trimmed. If you want to wear nail polish it must be clear.

  - Please bring your own make-up.

  - Please wear dark socks and dark, flat, comfortable shoes.

  - If you are cast as a manager, because of the shirt, please wear a flesh-colored bra (to match your skin).

Men - Your hair must be neatly trimmed. Your hair must be off your collar and trimmed up around your ears.

  - No facial hair.

  - Your nails must be clean and neatly trimmed.

  - Please bring your own make-up.

  - Please wear dark socks and dark, flat, comfortable shoes.

(More tips on back page.)

Sc 2525   CREW ROOM. ROBIN leaving room with hats and birthday
          stuff.

Sc 2530   KITCHEN. CAMERA FOLLOWS RHODA as she walks through
          quickly, coat and sunglasses on. She stops next to
          SALLY, the Production Caller.

                         RHODA
               Sally?

Sc 2530   CU SALLY

                         SALLY
               I heard. Birthday Party. Seven kids.
               Got it covered.

                         RHODA
               Thanks, you're terrific!

Sc 2540   SIDE LOBBY. JACK tells story to the KIDS, now wearing
          birthday hats. The birthday stuff is out. MRS.
          KOWALSKI and JACKIE watch, amused.

                         JACK
               And the other day I said to him, "Ron,"
               that's what I call him: "Ron," I said,
               "Ron, how come you wear such big
               shoes?" And this is what he told me.

In background we see RHODA fly out store.

Sc 2550   FRONT COUNTER. ROBIN assembles food (Happy Meal Boxes)
                          for the party.

Sc 2555   SIDE LOBBY. JACK continues to tell story. (JACKIE is
not in this scene.

                         JACK
               And he said, "That's right, Jack.
               And not only that," he said, "but
               I've got so much room inside my
               shoes that I've got an entire
               family of hamsters living in the
               left one, and lately they've been
               complaining about the squeak!"
               (the kids laugh)

ROBIN enters with the food.

myself and Jason and asked where he would want us to set our things. Sometimes we have a large area and sometimes a very small area, depending on where the shoot is being held. We have been in everything from large picture-perfect, gorgeous homes and studios, down to places not even worth mentioning. This first job site was an empty floor of a downtown Chicago building, which had been set up for this particular commercial. Several baby boys and girls were present. When children are under the age of three, producers often request "back ups," extra actors in case the children do not cooperate. Soon after we arrived, the producer chose which clothes Jason would be wearing from the selection I had brought. I'll never forget the shirt he picked. *Miami Vice,* a popular show then, which starred Don Johnson who often wore colorful floral shirts. That is the type of shirt the producer picked for Jason to wear in the commercial; a bright yellow Hawaiian one. He called him his "Miami Vice baby."

As far as I knew at that point, all of the babies had been hired as extras, except one little girl, who was considered a principal. A "principal," is one of the main characters who will be in close camera view. I was under the impression that the cutest babies are chosen as principals, but I found out that's not always true.

The producer started with the principal baby girl and a group of five babies. The kids were supposed to play with toys on a carpet while the adult principal spoke his lines. The producer wanted one baby on the go, and, since Jason was the most mobile on his knees, he was chosen to crawl from one end of the stage to the other when "action" was called. I did not know it at the time, but in the end, Jason was upgraded from an extra to a principal because he was in front of the camera, rather than being in the background. I'll explain later why this was such a nice bonus.

At least a hundred times, Jason crawled across that stage, but even to the last crawl he did it with a smile. He even amazed me. We broke for lunch and the mothers fed their children and gave them a nap if necessary. We have gone to what seemed to be high budget shoots in Chicago where, during breaks and lunch, all the food and drink was provided for everyone. Since this is not always the case, I suggest you bring your own food, unless you are told in advance that food will be available.

After lunch, it was time to start again. The producers were going to try using the babies who had not been on the set yet. I remember one gorgeous little baby girl with beautiful blue eyes and a perfect round face. Her mother put her on the stage and walked away. The little girl started crying. Mom returned and picked her up and she stopped crying. A few minutes later, they tried again, but the same thing happened. The producer said, "We'll try again later, because she is really so cute." They did, but that gorgeous baby girl would not cooperate. Although there are sometimes exceptions, it seems that no matter how cute children are, if they won't cooperate, or take directions well, the producers cannot use them. So the producer said, "Thanks, Mom, but no sense in staying," and released her. Later, I certainly came to know how that mom felt (as you'll see in Chapter Six, under "Don't Be a Stage Parent").

When the day was over and it was a final wrap, we were all so excited on the set because everything had gone so well. As it turned out, by being upgraded from an extra to a principal in a union commercial, Jason was paid residuals for several months. Not a bad way to start in this business! Plus there is more.

The next day Jason was asked to visit the photographer who was shooting the advertising for the print ads to accompany the union commercial. The photo shoot did not pay at the union rate (print work is not governed by the union) but it was a good hourly rate nonetheless, which was another bonus for us. The photo shoot was the following day, but guess what? Jason was a totally different baby. As soon as I put him down with two other babies who were in the commercial, he cried and cried. Now here was a challenging situation! Jason was already in the commercial shot the day before and the producer wanted the print ads to feature the same babies as the commercial had. I finally had to turn Jason's back toward the camera so you could not see him crying. You could still tell it was Jason because he had on the same clothes on. What an experience! It just goes to show how unpredictable babies are. Since it was our first job and Jason was already in the commercial, it would not bother me too much that he did not cooperate for the photo shoot. But in Chapter Six, under "Don't Be a Stage Mom," you will read about a different reaction from someone who thought she never would become a stage mom, and that stage mom was me!

Pay and Vouchers

Now that we have completed our first job how do we get paid? At the end of each print work job—newspaper, catalogue, magazine advertisement etc. and any non-union commercial work—I have to fill out a voucher for the agency that sent us (see sample). I will discuss union paperwork later in this chapter, which is entirely different. In the case of Jason's first job, I had to do both, fill out the agency voucher the second day for the photo shoot and fill out union paperwork on the day of the shoot. Each agency has its own type of voucher. The vouchers are at the job or the agency will send them to you in advance. Some are very simple, and some have wording that I must pay close attention to or I will be signing all my boys' rights aways (see Model's Release on voucher). The vouchers are usually filled out by the person in charge of the shoot, or he or she tells me the necessary information and I do it. The person in charge has to sign the voucher, and I sign on behalf of my sons because they are minors.

The vouchers usually have either three carbon copies: One goes to the studio; one goes to the agency; and I keep one for my files. The agency needs a copy of the voucher in order to bill out the job my son worked for. Usually, it is the advertising agency, but not always. Agency staff can become upset if you don't send those vouchers to them as soon as possible. I really can't blame them; they want to be paid too. Some of the talent agencies want you to send self-addressed stamped envelopes to make it convenient to send the check out faster. Others will send you a postcard letting you know they have your check and providing directions for you to follow. Agency fees range from fifteen to twenty percent for print work and non-union commercial work (depending on where you live) and ten percent for union commercial work. This is when talent agencies receive their pay. The checks should go directly to the agency, not always does it happen that way though. Once a check came directly to my home, which was highly unusual. I knew the agency was supposed to receive a commission, so I called them and then sent the commission.

As stated earlier, only union work is price regulated; just about anything else is negotiated between the talent agency staff and the advertising company. And every job is treated differently. One job might offer an hourly rate if the prints stay

Job Vouchers

MODEL'S RELEASE № 4058

MODEL			RATE
FITTING DATE	TIME FROM ___ TO		AMOUNT
JOB DATE	TIME FROM ___ TO		AMOUNT

● Chicago, Ill. 60611 ● 312-

INVOICE TO	REMARKS
ADDRESS	Billboards ☐
	National Ad ☐
CITY, STATE & ZIP CODE	Point of Purchase ☐
	Product Packaging ☐
ATT'N OF	Bonus to be paid $ _____

	TOTAL
STUDIO	15% S.C.
CLIENT	TOTAL
PRODUCT	JOB No.

INCOMPLETE VOUCHERS WILL NOT BE ACCEPTED

THIS RELEASE NOT VALID UNTIL PAYMENT IN FULL RECEIVED BY

_____   _____
CLIENT'S SIGNATURE   MODEL'S SIGNATURE

White & Yellow-Agency   Pink-Client   Gold-Model

13964

MODEL		RATE	
FITTING DATE	TIME FROM ___ TO		AMOUNT
JOB DATE	TIME FROM ___ TO		AMOUNT
INVOICE TO	P.O. JOB NO.	THIS TOTAL SUBJECT TO SERVICE CHARGE	TOTAL
ADDRESS	STUDIO		S.C. 15%
CITY/STATE/ZIP	CLIENT		
ATTN. OF	PRODUCT	REMARKS	

MODEL'S RELEASE

In consideration of the sum stated hereon. I hereby sell, assign and grant to above or those for whom they are acting as indicated above, the right and permission to copyright and/or use and/or publish photographic portraits or pictures of me in which I may be included in whole or in part or composite or reproductions thereof in color or otherwise made through print media at their studios or elsewhere for art advertising, trade or any other similar lawful purpose whatsoever, excluding television use.

I hereby waive my right to inspect and/or approve the finished product or the advertising copy that may be used in connection therewith.

I hereby release and discharge the above, its successors and all persons acting under its permission or authority or those for whom it is acting from any liability by virtue of any blurring, distortion, optical illusion or use in composite form that may occur or be produced in the taking of said picture or in any processing lending toward completion of the finished product.

THIS RELEASE NOT VALID UNTIL PAYMENT IN FULL RECEIVED BY

CLIENT X _____

MODEL X _____

THIS RELEASE TAKES PRECEDENCE OVER ANY RELEASE SIGNED AT THE TIME OF JOB WITH THE EXCEPTION OF CONTRACTS AND AGENCY RELEASES THAT CONTAIN THE SAME INFORMATION HEREIN.

Photography to be used for any of the following uses must be checked below, or the release is not valid.

☐ BILLBOARDS   ☐ POINT OF PURCHASE

☐ NATIONAL AD   ☐ PRODUCT PACKAGING

BONUS TO BE PAID $ _____ (AMOUNT) IF AD RUNS

LENGTH OF TIME AD WILL RUN _____

TERMS: NET 30 DAYS

INCOMPLETE VOUCHERS WILL NOT BE ACCEPTED

INVOICE DATE
FITTING AMOUNT
JOB AMOUNT
OTHER AMOUNT
TOTAL SUBJECT TO AGENCY FEE
AGENCY FEE
EXPENSES

TOTAL DUE THIS INVOICE ▶

TALENT LIABILITY RELEASE

_____ Productions,
is producing a series of commercials for _____ MARKETS
on February 12-13, 1992.

For the protection of _____ Productions and yourself, it is
necessary that you read and sign the following liability release.

By signing below, and for the consideration of $75ᵖᵉʳ ʰʳ, I do hereby give my consent and
authorization to _____ Productions, his immediate client, successors
and assigns, an irrevocable and unlimited right to use:

1. Any motion or still picture, or reproduction thereof, of me; or

2. Any recording, or reproduction thereof, of my voice, without
   further compensation to me. I hereby release _____
   Productions, its successors and assigns from all claims,
   liabilities, and damages from the use and/or reproduction
   of such materials.

It is understood that, _____ shall have the full and exclusive right
to such materials in any manner whatsoever. _I must be notified when using
other than Daane's markets._

X _Susan M. Halter_

Name _Jason Halter_
Address _____
City _____ State _____ Zip __-__

If the talent is a minor, Parent or Guardian must sign

I, the undersigned, being parent or guardian of the minor whose name appe
hereby consent to the foregoing conditions and warrant that I have the aut
to give such consent.

X _Susan M. Halter_ Name _Susan M_

_Susie —
Here you go.
Thanks for helping
us out! Hope to
work with you all
again soon!
Kev
P.S. The footage will only be used
for Daane's._

72

CONSENT AND RELEASE

FOR AND IN CONSIDERATION of the sum of _____ and other good and valuable consideration, receipt of which is hereby acknowledged, I do hereby, in behalf of myself, my heirs, executors, and administrators, sell, grant, assign, and deliver _____ its successors, agents, licensees, and assigns, all my right, title, and interest in and to all photographs, negatives, prints, paintings, drawings, sketches, and other reproductions of any kind now or hereafter made of me by _____ at its studios or elsewhere, and also the right to copyright, use, reproduce, license, display, retouch, alter, distort, caricature, publish, dispose of, and/or use in any other way _____ or any part of said photographs, negatives, prints, paintings, drawings, sketches, and other reproductions, with or without using my name, and/or with or without changes, distortions, or alterations thereon or additions thereto, and/or with or without display of any testimonial copy or any other form of advertising or display whatsoever used in connection therewith, regardless of whether the same is true or false, and/or with the name or names of any real or fictitious person or persons, or in any other manner whatsoever, including, but not by way of limitation, promotional, or training meetings of _____ agents, or representatives, or at meetings designed to recruit new sales people or employees for _____ or for use by _____ in their literature and advertising and/or for any other like or similar purpose. I specifically waive and surrender any claim which I may now or hereafter have that use of such pictures, photographs, colored slides, or motion pictures, or other reproductions, paintings, drawings, sketches, or of any other type would constitute an invasion of my privacy.

Signed this _____ day of _____, 19 _____

Description of Work: e.g., Slide, Page #, Key #, Issue #

_____

_____

_____

_____

_____

_____

_____

_____
Model's Signature

_____
Model Print Name

_____
Social Security Number

_____
Address

_____
City/State

_____
Photographer Print Name

_____
Witness

_____
Auth. Agent or Guardian's Signature (If model is under 18 years)

302167   0-3736

local; you then receive pay only for those hours worked. Working in both the Chicago and West Michigan markets, I find that my agency representatives here have a hard time convincing the advertisers to pay my boys the rates in Michigan that they receive in the Chicago market, unless they request experienced children who have been in the field for a long time. Then the rate is not a problem. You are paid a minimum of one hour on a job whether you work a full hour or not. After that, you are paid by the quarter hour. Normally, you are not paid for the audition times. In Chicago, if I am asked to bring a variety of clothes for my boys and they end up wearing them on the job, I note it on the paperwork, and we are paid for the use of our clothes as well as being paid for the boys' work. Some producer's will pay your mileage as well.

In addition to the vouchers that we have to sign at the job, the producer may have us sign another release form, for example a Consent and Release or Talent Release (see samples). Before signing any paperwork like this, including the agency vouchers, read it completely and ask any questions you may have. Generally, the release states, that either the photographer, producer, production company as well as others may use any recording or reproduction of the talent without further consent and without further compensation past a particular date. As you can see from the samples some releases can get quite detailed.

You'll notice I use the word "usually" quite often. In this field each job is different from the next, with the exception of union jobs, which are more predictable. Again, I want to stress that in this book I describe how things usually run, but, not always!

Keeping Track of the Paperwork

In the back of this book I have set up a Audition/Job Information Sheet to transfer all your information to from the carbon telephone pad by your telephone. Feel free to copy this page and put in a three ring binder. Sometimes it takes months to get paid for a certain job if it's not union. This helps keep paperwork organized. It is easy to forget if your child has been paid or not when there have been several jobs. When the job is completed and I have vouchers that need to be sent in when I return home, I immediately take care of sending the agency's voucher section to the agency with a self-addressed, stamped envelope. One time, I did not send a self-addressed envelope and the agency did not send Jason's check; it just sat in my son's file at the agency until I finally called to ask about our payment. After sending an envelope, I received Jason's check, but then I had to send it back because the check was voided after 90 days, and 90 days had passed. So I had to wait longer still for a new check to be issued. Do you see how important sending in that self-addressed stamped envelope is? All paperwork that pertains either to a audition or actual job is then attached to the call/job sheet. Once we are paid, to sheet is moved to the back of the book.

Union Pay

At Jason's first job, the healthcare insurance company, one person at the commercial shoot handled all of the union contracts. I am sorry to say that the company that holds the copyrighted contract forms that are filled out in order to receive payment, refused to grant me permission to reprint one of Jasons' contracts for this book. Reading a contract would be instructive for someone starting out. My experience in Chicago with the union commercials was that the check was sent directly to the agency, naming only Jason or Nicholas (whomever did the job) on the check, in care of the agency. In turn, the agency would send me a postcard (see sample), stating that they had received Jason's check and that I must send in their ten percent commission with a self-addressed, stamped envelope before they would send the paycheck to us. If they did not use this system, they would have to send the check to us and wait for us to send them their ten percent, probably not a favorable situation for them. In the event an exclusive agreement is signed between the talent and the talent agency, it may state that the talent agency has permission to endorse any checks issued in the talents name and take their commission and send on the difference to the talent.

We are holding a check for you at

Gross amount___366.60_____

Commission due_36.66___

Please come by and pick it up
or send us a self addressed
stamped envelope along with
your commission payment
                1S40A
Pickup times are: TUESDAY through FRIDAY
NO PICKUPS from noon to 2:00 PM

Postcard sent by talent agency notifing talent check has arrived for work performed. This is when the talent agency collects their fee!

CHAPTER 6

Guiding Your Child's Career: Learning About Unions, Self Promoting, Being a Stage Parent, and More...

Union or Non-Union—Is There a Difference?

In the previous chapter, I introduced the topic of union versus non-union employment, but I will discuss it in depth in this chapter. The pay for non-union commercials is not regulated as it is for union commercials. It is whatever the talent agency and the other parties involved (the advertising agency or the producer) agree to for a particular job. Usually, we are paid for the day's work on the set and nothing after the day of filming, which means no residuals. That is, no matter how many times a commercial runs, unless the paperwork states differently, we won't be paid anymore for the work.

Nicholas was called, without an audition, to appear in a commercial for a kids' play area in a local mall. The commercial was to air on the FOX network out of Grand Rapids. We spent approximately forty-five minutes from start to finish filming in a local home, with Nicholas wiping his feet and saying, "I'm wiping my feet, Mom." His pay at the time was sixty-five dollars for the shoot and, because it was a non-union job, that was it. That commercial has been running for eight months and still is at the time of this writing. Appearing in a commercial that runs over and over again is great exposure, but, at sixty-five dollars, and no further compensation, it was not one of Nicholas' higher paying jobs. Non-union jobs do not always provide low remuneration. They can be quite rewarding. It is important to remember that non-union jobs do not have a regulated pay scale as do union jobs. That is the nature of non-union work. The decision is yours as to whether you want to accept a non-union job, as long as you are not a member of the union.

As stated earlier, Jason's first commercial was a union regional commercial which paid him residuals. His pay as an extra that day was one-hundred twenty-five dollars. However, after the commercial was edited and ready to be aired, I was notified that Jason had been upgraded from an extra to a principal character because his face appeared up front in the camera for the final commercial, allowing him to receive a higher union scale instead of the extra's fee that was being paid to others.

I had to go back to the agency in Chicago which booked the commercial in order to sign the Standard Screen Actors Guild Employment Contract for Television Commercials, so that Jason could receive his payment as a principal character rather than as an extra. Union scale rate at that time was paid, and I was told that if the commercial were renewed every three months, he would receive another paycheck (residual). In addition, the commercial had been split into two commercial spots, a thirty-second and a fifteen-second spot. If both were renewed for a thirteen-week period (which is what a renewal period is) two checks would be issued to him. So, a job that had started out paying one-hundred twenty-five dollars when he was hired as an extra, turned out to be quite rewarding for Jason's future. And that was at the ripe old age of nine months! As of this writing, both boys had been under the Taft-Hartley law regarding unions. Taft-Hartley provides for a grace period of thirty days from the date of a person's first union commercial before he or she has to join the union. As soon as the thirty days have passed and the talent receives a call for another union commercial, he or she must join before accepting the work. Or if one's first job with the union runs over thirty days, one must join as well. Let me explain that last point further. After Jason's first commercial for the healthcare company in Iowa was edited, he was upgraded from an extra character to a principal, which increased his pay scale as well. With this union job, the Taft-Hartley law went into effect. In Nicholas' union situation, the table was turned a bit. When he was called for his first union commercial spot, he ended up being completetely edited out. Nicholas had done very well at the audition just the day before, but the next day at the shoot, he was a different person and would not cooperate. It was like night and day! Although the producer was surprised by the over-night difference in eighteen-month-old Nicholas, he said he was used to the startling behavior changes of little children. That is why back-up talent is hired.

Well, lo and behold, I received a depressing notice, addressed to Nicholas: "You have been completely edited out of the commercial." The commercial Nicholas was filmed for was a spot for a New York HMO, a major market. To my surprise, Nicholas still was paid for the day (a session fee) at the then-current union rate of three-hundred sixty-six dollars and sixty cents. That was all—no residuals. If Nicholas had been, at the time of this commercial, already under Taft-Hartley, and past his thirty days, he would have had to join the union for the then-current fee of nine-hundred four dollars and fifty cents. In union commercials, especially for national or major regional markets, the cost to join the union can be offset by the pay that the residuals provide every thirteen weeks.

Once a person is a union member, he or she cannot, or should not, audition for non-union work, which can be both good and bad. I have been informed that there is no question regarding an agency's responsibility to communicate clearly with its talent regarding union and non-union regulations. After all, a performer entrusts a talent agency with his or her professional care. Knowing who is and who is not union before sending the talent on auditions or jobs is of utmost importance. When a union job is in the process of being booked and the talent has been chosen, it is the producer's responsibility to inquire about the status of the talent and the responsibility of the union to respond to the producer's inquiry. The talent also has the responsibility for asking if the booking is a union or non-union job, just in case the personnel at one's agency is not familiar with the shoot and does not relay all of the necessary information. One can never ask enough questions. It is important to write down everything you are told regarding any audition or job, to refer to, if need be, at a later date.

Not all agencies are franchised with the union, nor do they have to be. But union-franchised agencies were what I looked for in the beginning, to find reputable agencies. Once in the business, you get a feel for the agencies and can tell who is reputable and who is not, whether they are union or non-union. A non-union booking rate can be lower, the same, similiar, or even higher than union pay rates; it just depends on how the job is negotiated.

Please take time to read the following text reprinted from the SAG brochure "Acting in Your Best Interest" for additional information about unions. Read also the other information provided by SAG. Many thanks to the Screen Actors Guild for granting me permission to reprint this valuable material. It shows they care about informing the public, too.

28

SCREEN ACTORS GUILD
5757 Wilshire Boulevard
Los Angeles, California 90036-3600

ACTING IN YOUR INTEREST

9 7
SCREEN ACTORS GUILD

81

Top Wages and Residual Payments

SAG basic contracts — which are negotiated with film, television and commercial producers — provide excellent minimum wages for the contemporary actor. The current film and TV scale is well over $400 a day. Guild contracts also provide payments for location work, overtime, holidays, travel time, mileage, stunts and wardrobe. In addition to these basic wages, the Guild has won residual payments in perpetuity for the re-use of all current films, TV shows and TV commercials. Last year, residual payments to SAG performers in all fields totalled $393 million. Since the inception of residuals in 1952, SAG has collected and distributed nearly $1.5 billion in film and TV show re-use fees in 8.5 million separate payments to performers. Commercial residuals have exceeded even that impressive total. Actors' salaries and economic clout continue to grow each year under Guild guidance.

Excellent Working Conditions

SAG contracts require certain comforts and amenitites during the production that enable performers to do their best work. Among the requirements established by the Guild are first class air travel with flight insurance, private dressing rooms, good meals and meal breaks, and adequate rest time between calls. Our contracts also require strict safety precautions and first aid on the set, special protections and education for minors, arbitration of disputes and grievances, collection of claims, and affirmative action in auditions and hiring. These working conditions are constantly monitored and enforced by SAG's professional staff. Without the Guild, these vital protections would not be in place today.

Pension and Health Plans

One of the primary benefits of working under SAG contracts is participation in the Screen Actors Guild — Producers Pension and Health Plans. Performers who earn a minimum SAG income of $5,000 a year are automatically enrolled for 12 months in the health Plan. Effective January 1, 1993 the Health Plan has two different levels, called Plan I and Plan II. Your covered earnings and previous years of Health Plan eligibility determine which Plan you qualify for. Both of these Plans cover your spouse and your dependent children.

If you earn $5,000 or more, you earn one Pension Credit for each calendar year in which you earn $5,000 ($2,000 a year prior to January 1, 1992) in SAG employment. Once you have earned 10 Pension Credits you become vested and qualify for a pension upon retirement. There are currently some 3,600 SAG pensioners who receive monthly payments ranging from a minimum of $220 to a maximum of $4,000, depending on past income.

These valuable benefits are paid entirely by the employer — SAG members do not contribute to the Pension and Health Plans. Every time a performer works under a SAG contract, the producer pays 12.65% above the base salary to Pension and Health in order to provide these benefits. Previously qualified members whose earnings fall below the $5,000 eligibility level can enroll in the "self-pay program" to maintain medical insurance for up to 18 months. Pension and Health benefits are governed by a Board of trustees composed of equal numbers of actors' and producers' representatives. Complete benefit booklets are available free of charge from all Pension and Health Offices:

SCREEN ACTORS GUILD — PRODUCERS' PENSION and HEALTH PLANS

NATIONAL HEADQUARTERS — Hollywood
5757 Wilshire Boulevard
Los Angeles, California 90036-3600
(213) 465-4600

New York
1515 Broadway, 44th Floor
New York, New York 10036
(212) 382-1020

Chicago
307 North Michigan Avenue, Suite 1005
Chicago, Illinois 60601
(312) 372-3749

Democratic Participation

The collective wisdom, experience and energy of our members are the Guild's greatest assets. Among the primary privileges of SAG membership are the right to vote in Guild elections and contract ratifications, join in membership meetings, serve on committees and run for Guild office. Using these democratic methods, the principles of the Guild are devised through debate and majority rule. Your Guild vote is your voice in the shape and direction of your profession.

Casting Contacts and Assistance

While the Guild does not secure employment for members, it does provide some extremely valuable casting assistance for those who may wish to employ you. Our Agency Registry staff gives the name and phone number of your agent or designated business contact to all SAG-signatory production personnel who are trying to reach you. As a SAG member, you can always be located by a potential employer, even if you don't currently have an agent.

The Guild also maintains wide-ranging Skills & Talent Survey of members, so that casting directors seeking specific abilities can quickly locate all members with those desired skills. The Survey covers 300 languages from Arabic to Zulu, and more than 150 special talents from acrobatics to yodeling. Our computer can cross-reference all these skills, thus enabling a casting director to identify a member who can simultaneously surf and speak Spanish, for example, or any other combination of abilities.

Several Guild branches publish local talent directories of members for distribution throughout the casting community. In addition, some Guild branches sponsor free talent showcases and seminars with agents and casting directors. A few of the larger Guild branches also provide telephone casting information hotlines for members, and post current production charts and casting contacts on bulletin boards in Guild offices.

In New York and Hollywood, the Guild sponsors special affirmative action employment access programs for performers of color and performers with disabilities. In these programs, the Guild secures the agreement of local commercial casting directors and advertising agencies to conduct general interviews, to attend Guild-sponsored talent showcases, and to accept photos and resumes from members in these protected groups.

Talent Agency Franchsing

SAG provides a wide range of protections for members in their dealings with talent agents. Nationwide, some 500 agencies are currently franchised by the Guild to represent its members. To secure a SAG franchise, talent agents must sign a 75-page agreement known as the SAG Agency Regulations. These rules require ethical conduct and state licenses (where applicable), among other conditions. One of the Guild's primary regulations strictly limits agents' commissions to 10% of actors' salaries. The SAG rules also allow members to terminate agency contracts for cause, and offer several other advantages not shared by non-union performers and unregulated agents. SAG agents cannot send Guild members on non-union auditions, nor can agents cast, produce or act in any SAG motion pictures.

Craft Programs and Seminars

Nearly all SAG branches offer an assortment of craft programs and seminars designed to enhance members' skills and professionalism. The SAG Conservatory, offered in most regions, is a very inexpensive alternative to the costly classes that are commercially available. The Conservatory conducts training sessions in on-camera and audition skills, and frequently invites well-known guests to address members on the craft of acting. Several Guild branches also offer free seminars and showcases with local agents and casting directors.

In Hollywood and New York, the Guild sponsors SAG Film Societies where members can, for a small annual membership fee, attend private screenings of the best current films with an audience of fellow performers. These craft-enhancement programs are among SAG's most popular membership services, and generally fill up early.

Credit Unions and Financial Services

A full range of financial services is available to SAG members through two federally-insured credit unions designed just for performers. The AFTRA-SAG Federal Credit Union, headquarterd in Hollywood with additional offices in Chicago and Florida, serves performers throughout the United States except in New York, where members are served by the Actors Federal Credit Union. Both of these financial institutions are overseen by quafied actor-trustees and offer low-cost loans, high-yield savings, free checking accounts, credit cards, payroll deduction programs, even a special saving plan for residuals. Best of all, the credit unions are owned by their members, and all profits are returned to share-holders through quarterly dividends.

AFTRA-SAG Federal Credit Union
6922 Hollywood Boulevard, Suite 304
Hollywood, Californa 90028
(213) 461-3041
In California (800) 354-3728
In the Continental U.S. (800) 826-6946

AFTRA-SAG Federal Credit Union
75 East Wacker Drive, Suite 1700
Chicago, Illinois 60601
(312) 553-1924

AFTRA-SAG Federal Credit Union
2041 NW 2nd Avenue
North Miami, Florida 33169
(305) 770-9206

Actors Federal Credit Union
165 West 46th Street, 14th Floor
New York, New York, 10036
(212) 869-8926

Publications and Merchandise

The Guild publishes an award-winning national magazine, *Screen Actor*, as well as regional branch newsletters to inform members about issues and events in their local markets and the industry as a whole. In addition to these periodicals, the Guild produces a number of free booklets of interest to members, such as *The Young Performer's Handbook, The Actor's Guide to California Unemployment Benefits, On-the-Set Safety Bulletins* and more. The Guild also publishes a highly useful Professional Calendar/Organizer which is sold to members at a nominal fee. An attractive line of SAG-logo merchandise is also available for purchase by members.

Free Income Tax Assistance

The United States Internal Revenue Service trains volunteer Guild members to assist fellow performers in preparing and filing annual income tax returns. This is a free service offered to qualified members each year in New York, Hollywood and Chicago.

College Scholarships

Through the independent, non-profit Screen Actors Guild Foundation, SAG members and their children can apply for a John Dales Scholarship to attend an accredited institution of higher learning. The Foundation is now developing several educational programs to benefit members and the acting profession in the future.

Benevolent Funds and Social Services

The SAG Foundation also administers the Guild's Emergency Assistance Fund which helps qualified members in dire financial need. Guild members may also become eligible for financial assistance and other social services through the Actors Fund of America, the Motion Picture Players Welfare Fund and the Motion Picture & Television Fund.

Housing

The Guild is actively involved in the development and management of affordable housing for SAG members in the two largest acting markets. In New York, members may become eligible to live at the low-cost Manhattan Plaza Apartments. In Hollywood, the Guild is a founding participant in Housing for Entertainment Professionals, a coalition of performing arts unions seeking to establish low-cost apartments for performers in greater Los Angeles.

Qualified senior members may also be eligible for residence in one of two retirement homes for the entertainment industry, although there are waiting lists for admission. The Actors Fund operates a retirement and nursing home for actors in New Jersey, and the Motion Picture & Television Fund runs a retirement home and hospital in Los Angeles for all film industry workers.

Retraining and Re-employment

Guild members may take advantage of two professional retraining programs jointly sponsored with other performers' unions. The Career Transition for Dancers program helps counsel and retrain performers who are retiring from dance, and the Actors' Work program provides similar services for senior performers and others with special needs. The SAG Foundation will soon be expanding services in this area as well.

Community and Legislative Advocacy

The Guild is often called upon by members to assist in non-partisan community and legislative matters that directly affect performers. Guild branches frequently work with regional film commissions to help encourage local production. Guild officers and executive use their influence with local, state and national legislators to advance legal solutions to performers' concerns. Among the Guild's legislative victories are: performers' exemptions under federal income tax reform, non-discriminatory auto insurance rates for actors, celebrities' image rights after death, confidentiality of home addresses, and defense of First Amendment rights, such as artistic freedom from censorship. In the public arena, the Guild often serves as the unified voice of the screen acting community.

Networking and Social Events

Guild branches sponsor a wide array of special events each year, from round table discussions to award presentations to picnics. These activities allow members to network with fellow performers and others in the local production community, such as agents, casting directors and producers. Some of these events are educational in purpose, others are designed simply for social enjoyment and solidarity among SAG performers.

A Helping Hand

No matter what your needs as a member, the Screen Actors Guild is ready to assist you. If you need help on the set, the Guild will dispatch a representative to assess the problem. If you need to file a claim or grievance against an employer, the Guild is there to defend your rights. If you need information, our staff will gladly answer general questions and give you practical advice about the realities of your local market. If you're interested in networking with fellow actors and industry professionals, the Guild has a caucus, committee or special event for you. Membership in the Screen Actors Guild is a very valuable tool in a performing arts career. Make the most of it.

A Shared Vision

In 1933, a small but brave group of actors founded a new craft guild to represent performer's interests in the burgeoning film industry. Nearly 60 years later, the Screen Actors Guild is still representing actors' interests in a worldwide entertainment industry that SAG's founders never imagined. Although the business has changed dramatically, our founders' goals and ideals are still being pursued by the Guild and its members today.

Performers created SAG to bring dignity and respect to the professional screen actor, to guarantee a living wage and a safe, supportive working environment where the performing arts can flourish. through self-government and collective bargaining with motion picture producers, the Guild has created a new atmosphere — and a whole new range of benefits — for film and TV performers. These ongoing benefits are among the many advantages of membership in the Screen Actors Guild.

We Are the Professionals

Membership in SAG says that you are an experienced, professional screen actor. Our ranks include the world's finest actors, stunt performers, insgers, voice performers, dancers, extras, pilots and puppeteers. As professionals, we have established certain minimum standards that must be met in order for us to give our best performances — that's why we don't do non-union work. We pride ourselves on being the best talent available, and for that reason producers seek us out and sign our basic agreements. The 60-year history of the Guild is the story of our advancement from easily-exploitable outcasts to highly admired artists.

By the Member, For the Member

The Guild is not "them," it is "us." SAG is a representative democracy run by members, for members. And it is more than a trade union — it is our collective voice in the future of our profession and our industry. Our strength is founded in unity of purpose, mutual support and common concern for the needs of our difficult profession.

The Guild is governed by a national Constitution and By-Laws which have been written, adopted and enforced by performers for the greater good of the whole membership. The highest policy-making body of the Guild is the National Board of Directors, which is elected by the membership, from the membership. All members in good standing for at least two years are eligible to run for the Board, and any member may serve on its many advisory committees where Guild policies are hammered out through democratic debate. SAG officers are all volunteers and are not paid for their service.

SAG business is also conducted through local branch councils, open membership meetings and confidential mail votes. Guild services are financed primarily by members' dues and initiation fees, which are established by a vote of the membership.

NATIONAL HEADQUARTERS
Screen Actors Guild
5757 Wilshire Boulevard
Los Angeles, California 90036-3600

MAIN SWITCHBOARD . . . .(213) 465-4600
Actors to locate . . . .(213) 549-6737
Agency . . . .(213) 549-6745
Commercials/Music Video . . . .(213) 549-6858
Industrial/Educ. Contracts . . . .(213) 549-6847
Television Contracts . . . .(213) 549-6835
Theatrical Contracts . . . .(213) 549-6828
Production Services . . . .(213) 549-6811
Singers' Representative . . . .(213) 549-6864
Communications . . . .(213) 549-6654
Dues Information . . . .(213) 549-6755
Legal Affairs . . . .(213) 549-6627
Membership Services . . . .(213) 549-6770
Residuals . . . .(213) 549-6505
Signatory Records . . . .(213) 549-6869
Sta-12 (work Clearance) . . . .(213) 549-6794
SAG Foundation . . . .(213) 549-6709

NEW YORK HEADQUARTERS
Screen Actors Guild
1515 Broadway, 44th Floor
New York, New York 10036

MAIN SWITCHBOARD . . . .(212) 944-1030
Affirmative Action . . . .(212) 827-1433
Agency-member contacts and contracts . . . .(212) 944-6797
Committees . . . .(212) 827-1448
Membership Inquiry . . . . (212) 944-6243
Signatory Status-to check on company . . . .(212) 827-1470

WHAT ALL PERFORMERS SHOULD KNOW ABOUT AFTRA - SAG ...and the "BUSINESS"

A Handy Orientation Guide for new members and non-members by:

The American Federation of Television and Radio Artists
Screen Actors Guild

San Diego Local Branch
7827 Convoy Court Suite 400
San Diego, California 92111

(619) 278-7695
Casting Hotline: (619)278-2918

WHY THE INITIATION FEES?

Newcomers to the Union pay the one-time initiation fee to share in the cost of past negotiations in securing improved wages and benefits which new members enjoy at once. The initiation fee entitles an active member to all rights as a member of AFTRA and/or SAG anywhere in the nation, also giving you "portability"-the ability to move and transfer to other locals.

A FEW IMPORTANT RULES:

Rule 1-No Contract/No Work! This rule was enacted by the members themselves. It means you can be disciplined if you do a non-union job. When we can't enforce contracts, we can't collect wages or Health and Retirement or Pension monies.

Is your employer a signatory? Be sure to check with the local office to find out if the employer has signed to the appropriate contract under which you would perform BEFORE accepting employment. The office can assist in contacting the producer and have him/her sign to an agreement, either as a full-time signatory, or for one performance only.

AUDITONS. You may audition for any job. Feel free to contact the office about the employer's status. If they are not signatory, we can still contact them and answer any concerns or questions they may have about the union. In many instances, we have successfully persuaded producers that it is to their benefit as well as the performers' to work with a union contract.

Always be sure to file a member report after each and every job. This document is a contract, and it is the member's responsibility to fill it in, sign it and have your employer sign it. Ask the office for a member report, and examples of how to properly complete it. Always live up to the contract. Know your rights and obligations, and never accept work for less than scale. Remember, the contract is a two-way street.

ABOUT TALENT AGENTS

Union members may only be represented by those agents holding the applicable AFTRA and/or SAG franchise. In other words, if you are a member of AFTRA only, you may not be represented by an agent who is only SAG franchised. The office will provide you a list. Agents may not receive more than 10% commission on your gross earnings.

THE SIGNATORY MAZE

A signatory is a producer, studio or ad agency which has signed to one or more of the AFTRA-SAG Codes. Producers will sign because they want to hire YOU.YOU give them quality in the product, which makes them look good in the client's mind. YOU give them professionalism, save them valuable production time with one or two takes instead of fourty.

BEWARE OF SCAMS

Spend your hard earned money wisely. Check out the credentials of agents, acting coaches, and photographers. NEVER pay someone to line up auditions or acting opportunities. Do not to allow an agent to select their photographer for new pictures. Compare several prices of headshots and composites. Evaluate several photographers' work before the shoot. Find out from other talent if THEIR pictures produced results. Network with other union members and find out what's really happening.

OTHER BENEFITS

*Group legal Services   *Casting Hotline
*Theater Authority Fund *SAG Travel Serv.
*Dental Insurance   *Financial Aid
*Toll-free H&R, signatory hotlines
*Membership portability
* Free Grievance & Arbitration
Note: This booklet represents only an overview of the subjects contained within. For more details, call the local office.

WHY JOIN THE UNION?

1) The Union negotiates minimum scale wages and defines fair working conditions. If you are a member at one of television or radio stations KFMB AM-FM or TV, KCBQ, KSDO-AM, KFSD, or KPOP, the AFTRA contract guarantees vacations, holiday pay, sick leave and severance pay, as well as freedom from onerous hours, split shifts, unfair scheduling and unfair discharge. AFTRA and SAG's some 40 different contracts are the summation of over 50 years of arduous negotiation.

2) For freelancers, the Union collects wages, and handles all claims. Depending on which contract you perform under, you will be paid within a specified timeframe.

3) Union signatory employers (producers who sign to union agreements) pay into your Health and Retirement (Pension) fund. Check the current minimum annual earnings test under AFTRA or SAG to qualify for health insurance coverage, helping you pay your doctor and hospital bills.

4) Union signatory employers pay your residual (reuse) fees for commercial/program work.

5) NO MORE CATTLE CALLS! Union signatory employers are obligated to schedule you for specific interview/audition times and are responsible for paying you for any time spent over one hour on 1st and 2nd auditions, plus a fee for 3rd call-backs.

6) Union members work with union franchised talent agents who may negotiate for over scale, and they collect no more than 10% of your gross earnings.

7) The Union has membership meetings, a newsletter, and "Conservatory" workshop/seminar programs to keep you informed and help you learn more about the performing craft by keeping your "tools" sharp.

8) The Union offers the AFTRA-SAG credit union, featuring low interest loan and credit card services. Scholarships, financial aid, and several other benefits are available to union members. Ask the office for details.

9) The Union is run by members for its members. Union members have a voice within the democracy which governs their union and a vote that will be counted. Consider taking an interest by joining a committee, attending meetings, run for the AFTRA Board or SAG Council, and find out what it's really all about.

10) Union members on the average make more money than their non-union counterparts, according to a recent BNA study.

WHAT THE UNION IS NOT

The union is not a hiring hall, but assists its members in getting the kind of information they can use to get the jobs, via the union's casting hotline, signatory list, newsletter, and Conservatory events. And once you get the union job (when the producer signs to appropriate code), you are guaranteed protection under a contract with fair wages and benefits. Too many performers sell themselves short only to discover how much they find they need the union when they find they've been taken advantage of by their employer.

WHAT IS SAG?

Screen Actors Guild, affiliated with the AFL-CIO, represents 75,000 professional actors and performing artists nationwide working in motion pictures, including features, made-for television films, commercials, music videos, and student and educational projects produced on film.

HOW DO I JOIN SAG?

For principal performers with a speaking role, proof of employment or prospective employment under SAG contract, and for Extra players, a minimum of three work days after 3/25/90 with a signatory employer. A performer may join SAG if a paid up member of AFTRA, AEA, AGVA, AGMA or ACTRA for a period of at least one year AND has worked at least one principal job in the other union's jurisdiction. SEG members as of 12/1/89 may join SAG without proof of employment, provided they are paid-up.

The joining fees are   payable by bank check or money order. Appointments to join need to be made with the local membership administrator. Your application and qualifications for joining will be fully investigated, so please do not falsely represent your credentials.

WHAT IS AFTRA?

The American Federation of Television and Radio Artists is a nationwide union with 70,000 members and is associated with the AFL-CIO. Every performer who speaks, sings, dances or acts before the microphone or television camera as well as those engaged to make transcriptions, videotape commercials, phonograph recordings video cassettes, industrial videos or slide presentations recorded to audio or video tape should be a member of AFTRA.

HOW DO I JOIN AFTRA?

At present, AFTRA is an "open" union. Performers may simply join by tendering the appropriate dues and initiation fee of $865.00. Appointments to join should be made with the membership administrator in advance.

★ SCREEN ACTORS GUILD

★ NEW MEMBERSHIP INFORMATION ★

★ JOINING QUALIFICATIONS

A performer may become eligible for Screen Actors Guild membership under one of the following conditions:

1) PROOF OF SAG EMPLOYMENT

A. Principal Performer Employment

Performers may join SAG upon proof of employment or prospective employment within two weeks or less by a SAG signatory company. Employment must be in a principal or speaking role in a SAG film, videotape, television program or commercial. Proof of such employment may be in the form of a signed contract, a payroll check or check stub, or a letter from the company (on company letterhead stationery) The document proving employment must provide the following information: applicant's name and Social Security number, the name of the production or the commercial (the product name), the salary paid in dollar amount, and the specific date(s) worked.

B. Extra Players Employment

Performers may join SAG upon proof of employment as a SAG covered extra player at full SAG rates and conditions for a MINIMUM of three work days subsequent to March 25, 1990. Employment must be by a company signed to a SAG Extra Players Agreement, and in a SAG film, videotape, television program or commercial. Proof of such employment must be in the form of a signed employment voucher (or time card), plus a payroll check or check stub. Such documents must provide the same information listed in paragraph 1)A above.

2) Employment Under an Affiliated Performers' Union

A. Performers may join SAG if the applicant is a paid-up member of an affiliated performers' union (AFTRA, AEA, AGVA, AGMA or ACTRA) for a period of at least one year AND has worked at least once as a principal performer in that union's jurisdiction.

★ JOINING FEE: $1,122.50

To join SAG, a performer must pay an initiation fee of $1,080.00, plus the first semi-annual basic dues of $42.50, for a total joining fee of $1,122.50. All joining fees are payable in full, in cashier's check or money order, at the time of application. NO PERSONAL CHECKS are accepted for joining fees. Fees may be lower if you join in some branch areas, OR if you are a **paid-up member of an affiliated performers' union.**

★ LEGITIMACY OF APPLICATION

Your application and proof of employment will be fully investigated by the Guild. Your application for SAG membership will be denied if you have falsified your credentials, or if your qualifying employment is not bona fide. While it is your responsibility to ascertain the validity of your qualifying employment, the Guild will be the sole arbiter in determining whether the employer was legitimate or bogus, and whether the qualifying employment which you performed was actual production work or work created solely to enable you to gain Guild membership.

Please be aware that false representation or deception on your part will jeopardize your chances to join the Guild. Further, if after your application has been granted the Guild discovers such misconduct on your part, you may find yourself subject to disciplinary proceedings which could result in your being fined, suspended and/or expelled from the Guild.

★ APPOINTMENTS FOR ADMISSION

If you are eligible under the conditions stated above, please contact your nearest SAG office BEFORE COMING IN so we can advise you of the amount of your joining fee and arrange an appointment with the New Membership Department.

New Membership Department
SCREEN ACTORS GUILD

PROFILE ★ SCREEN ACTORS GUILD

★ Name & Affiliation

Screen Actors Guild (SAG), AFL-CIO. Chartered as part of the Associated Actors and Artistes of America (Four A's), which also includes the American Federation of Television and Radio Artists (AFTRA); Actors' Equity Association (AEA); The American Guild of Musical Artists (AGMA); and the American Guild of Variety Artists (AGVA). SAG is also a member of the International Federation of Actors (FIA), a global organization of performers' unions.

★ Size & Jurisdiction

SAG represents over 84,000 professional actors and performing artists working in motion pictures nationwide, including theatrical features and television films, prime time television programs, TV commercials, interactive multimedia productions, infomercials, industrial and educational films, student and experimental films, and music videos.

★ Our Members

SAG members work as principal performers, student performers, singers, dancers, extras, voice-over performers, pilots, puppeteers and models. Members range from infants to veteran performers more than 100 years old. Although our top stars are well paid, over 80% of SAG members earned $10,000 or less in the SAG jurisdiction last year, and the great majority of Guild members are unemployed as performers on any given day.

★ Geographic Spread

The Screen Actors Guild was founded in Hollywood, California, and approximately 46,000 performers are part of the general membership in greater Los Angeles today. New York is the second largest membership area with almost 25,000 members. Florida is third with 4,000 members, followed by Chicago with 3,000 and San Francisco with 2,500. SAG also maintains branches in Atlanta, Boston, the Carolinas, Dallas, Denver, Detroit, Honolulu, Houston, Las Vegas, Nashville, New Mexico, Philadelphia, Phoenix, San Diego, Utah and Washington, D.C. Members in other geographical areas are served through the national SAG office as well as local AFTRA offices.

★ Guild Government

SAG is a highly democratic union run by a National Board of Directors. Board members are all performers elected to three-year terms on a proportional, regional basis. The three nationally elected officers are President, Recording Secretary and Treasurer, all of whom must reside in the Los Angeles area. In addition, there are 12 National Vice Presidents elected regionally. All officers and Board members are elected by secret ballot, mailed to the entire paid-up membership. SAG regional branches have local officers and a local council in addition to their national representatives. The National Board of Directors is the highest policy-making body within the union, with interim decisions delegated to the Executive Committee, which is comprised of the 15 national officers and other members elected by the Board. All SAG officers are elected from the active membership, by the membership, and are not paid for their services.

Policies established by the Board of Directors are implemented and enforced on a day-to-day basis by a paid, professional staff headed by the National Executive Director in Hollywood.

★ President

Actor Richard Masur is well known to film and television audiences from his starring roles in the series, *One Day At A Time*, *Picket Fences*, *The Hot L Baltimore*, and *Rhoda*, as well as over thirty-five television films, four of which are among the top-ten rated T.V. movies of all time, including *Adam*, *Fallen Angel*, *When The Bough Breaks*. He also received an Emmy Nomination for his performance opposite Farrah Fawcett in *The Burning Bed*. He also was seen in the much heralded *And the Band Played On* for HBO and appeared as General Leslie Groves in *Hiroshima* on Showtime.

His over thirty-five feature films include *Under Fire*, *Risky Business*, *Heaven's Gate*, *Who'll Stop The Rain*, *Heartburn*, *The Believers*, *Shoot to Kill*, *Flashback*, *My Girl*, *My Girl 2*, *The Man Without a Face*, *Six Degrees of Separation*, *Les Patriotes*, *Forget Paris*, and *Multiplicity*.

Masur has moved from being a familiar face for over 20 years in film and television to directing. His first project, *Love Struck*, a 23-minute film which he both wrote and directed, was nominated for an Academy Award for Best Live Action Short Film. For his next effort, *Torn Between Two Fathers*, an After School Special, Masur was nominated for the prestigious Directors Guild of America Award. He has since directed multiple episodes of *The Wonder Years*, and an episode of *Picket Fences*.

★ Past Presidents

Former first officers of the Guild, starting in 1933, are: Ralph Morgan, Eddie Cantor, Robert Montgomery, Edward Arnold, James Cagney, George Murphy, Ronald Reagan, Walter Pidgeon, Leon Ames, Howard Keel, George Chandler, Dana Andrews, Charlton Heston, John Gavin, Dennis Weaver, Kathleen Nolan, William Schallert, Edward Asner, Patty Duke and Barry Gordon.

★ Officers

In addition to President Richard Masur, SAG's current national officers are F.J. O'Neil, Treasurer, and Kathy Connell, Recording Secretary. The 12 Regional Vice Presidents are: 1st VP (LA) Sumi Haru; 2nd VP (NY) Mel Boudrot; 3rd VP (LA) Daryl Anderson; 4th VP (NY) Kim Sykes; 5th VP (Chicago) Mary Seibel; 6th VP (SF) Scott DeVenney; 7th VP (Florida) Harold Bergman; 8th VP (Regional Branches) Lon Carli; 9th VP (LA) Kitty Swink; 10th VP (NY) Maureen Donnelly; 11th VP (LA) Amy Aquino; 12th VP (NY) Larry Keith. All national officers are elected to two-year terms.

★ Executive Staff

SAG's professional staff is headed by National Executive Director Ken Orsatti in Hollywood, and Associate National Executive Director John T. McGuire in New York City. They oversee a paid staff of nearly 300 employees nationwide, and serve as the Guild's chief contract negotiators. Each branch office is run by a local executive director.

★ Collective Bargaining

SAG's two major contracts with producers cover theatrical films and television programs, and TV commercials. The 1995 Basic Theatrical and Television Agreement, negotiated with the Alliance of Motion Picture and Television Producers, is effective through June 30, 1998. The 1994 Commercials Contract, negotiated with national advertisers and ad agencies, is in effect through 1997. Additional contracts cover interactive multimedia, industrial and educational films and videos, student films, Spanish language commercials, Public Broadcasting System productions, low-budget features and music videos.

★ Responsibilities

The Guild's primary responsibilities include: negotiating contracts which establish the minimum wages and working conditions for professional performers; enforcement of those contracts; processing residual payments to members (for re-use of films and TV shows); regulation and franchising of talent agents; membership record-keeping and communications. SAG does not secure employment for its members.

SAG strives to protect actors' wages and working conditions through aggressive advocacy at the bargaining table; representation on motion picture sets and locations; cooperative forums with employers; and increasingly, through legislative lobbying at the local, state and national levels.

SAG is also concerned with its members' general welfare and quality of living. Qualified members are provided with excellent medical insurance and a pension plan, established through collective bargaining with producers. The SAG-Producers Pension and Health Plan is jointly administered by labor and management, and has offices in Los Angeles, New York and Chicago.

SAG RULE ONE: Members are prohibited from working within SAG's jurisdiction for any producer who fails to sign a collective bargaining agreement with the Guild.

★ Historical Perspective

In 1933, when the Guild was formed, actors were lucky to be paid $15 for a long day's work or $66 for a 6-day week. Unregulated hours and working conditions were even worse than the pay. In March of that year, producers decreed a 50% pay cut for all actors under studio contracts. With no organization or collective bargaining power, the actors took the cut.

As a result of the producers' unilateral action, a small group of Hollywood actors met to consider forming a self-governing guild of motion picture actors, which would give performers a unified voice. Articles of Incorporation were filed in Sacramento on June 30, 1933, followed by a four year struggle for union recognition and a contract with producers.

In 1937, after affiliating with the American Federation of Labor, SAG's early members voted to strike if necessary to achieve union recognition. With over 95% of the major stars of the time ready to walk off the job, the producers acquiesced, and on May 9, 1937, SAG had its first contract governing wages and working conditions for actors in feature films.

Since then, through collective bargaining with producers, SAG has created a new working environment for motion picture performers. First established were regular working hours, meal periods, a five-day week, and premium pay for working overtime, Sundays, and holidays. Successive contracts have brought a multitude of continuing benefits to SAG members, including: increased wages for all performers, pension and health plans paid by the producer, residual payments for re-use of motion pictures, regulation of talent agents and their commissions, safety standards on the set, and affirmative action in hiring, among others.

★ Information

For more information on the history, organization and activities of the Screen Actors Guild contact the National Communications Department at Hollywood headquarters:

SCREEN ACTORS GUILD
5757 Wilshire Boulevard
Los Angeles, CA 90036-3600
(213) 549-6654

★ Guild Motto

"They best serve themselves who serve others."

92

Don't Be a Stage Parent

In Chapter Five, "The Day of the Job," I spoke of the beautiful little girl who just would not stop crying, and so the producer of the commercial could not use her. At the time I could not feel what her mother was going through. That was before Nicholas was edited out of the New York area commercial. I felt such heartbreak and realized afterwards I was indeed behaving like a stage mom. I hope every parent in this business will catch him- or herself when it first happens. I am glad I did, and I won't let it happen again.

The commercial was actually supposed to have been for Jason, but when I arrived and saw Nicholas' age group auditioning as well, I showed the producer his pictures and he said, "If you can get back here before we end the audition we will see him." We made it back in time. Nicholas, like Jason, had to walk on a balance beam and do somersaults on a gym mat and just loved it. A couple of hours after the audition, the talent agency called—Jason did not get the job but Nicholas did.

The shoot was held the next day; that terrific kid who did such a grand job of winning the heart of the producer would not even go near him, let alone walk on the balance beam. I just could not understand it. I then realized exactly how the mom in Jason's healthcare commercial felt. However, the producer was just great; he waited and used the others who had also been booked, and then came back to Nicholas twice. Nicholas was wearing blue jean cutoffs and had "such cute legs," I remember hearing the producer say. He really wanted to use him, but Nicholas still would not cooperate fully. They did get him to walk the beam, but I could see on the monitor that he really was not enjoying it. After the third try, the producer's assistant came out and gave me the word, "Sorry, we will have to release your son." He gave us the necessary union papers to fill out because this was a union job, and then said we could leave. We should have left, but didn't. I simply would not accept the fact that Nicholas did not want to do what he had done so well just one day earlier (a sign of a stage mom).

So, after we were released to go, I decided to stay, hoping the producer would try Nicholas just once more. Maybe he would change back into the same little guy of the day before. I did get what I wanted, the producer tried him one more time, since we were still there. But the results were the same. I could even see it in the other mothers' eyes: "Mom, just go home, he is not in the mood today." Not once did the producer or his assistant get angry with me, when, by rights, they could have and I would have deserved it.

Not until I returned home and started reading the literature provided by the producer who was shooting the commercial, did I realize how out of place I was. That producer works with children all the time and understands that kids, like adults, have bad days, too. In this business, such a sensitive quality in a person is special and rare. So, thank you, Mr. Bob Ebel, for bringing me to my senses without even knowing it. Remembering what it is like to be a kid can make all the difference in the world when a person deals with children. Now it all made sense why he and his staff had been so understanding. And I had behaved like a total stage mom, something I had told myself I would never do. How foolish I must have looked. This man understood my child better than I did! I learned that day if my kids cooperate, great; if they don't, that's all right too. You cannot and should not force a child to perform. I also learned from that point on, to believe that there will be another opportunity at another time for my child to shine.

Stage Parent, Part Two

I think another part of not being a stage mom, is avoiding being boastful about my boys' accomplishments. As I have said, doing this type of work is just another activity for them. And again, whether they get the commercial or not, they are still special. I don't talk about what they have done unless another person brings it up first. For a long time, most people around us, beyond our family, didn't know that Jason and Nicholas appear in commercials and advertisements. Then a close family friend told a fellow worker who was also a local newspaper reporter about Jason and Nicholas. The reporter was fascinated by what we do, and, thinking many readers would be as well, she asked if she could interview us for an article in the paper. I thought and thought about it. I just didn't know if I wanted the publicity for them but decided to say yes, so that maybe some of our experience could help others. The article was going to be in the back of the paper, in a small section called "Interesting Persons." How many people would see it, anyway?

Well, the editor thought it was such an interesting piece that he made it a front-page main story.

Later, I found out it did help one parent who had seen an ad in the paper for "MODELS," like the one I spoke of at the beginning of this book, and wanted to know whether she should respond to the ad. I felt good that I was able to shed some light on the industry for her. That's when the idea for this book started to come to life, along with other events in my life that pointed me in this direction.

At school, the day after the article came out, teachers were asking seven-year-old Jason for his autograph. He came home and asked, "Why are people asking me for my autograph, Mom, just because my picture was in the paper? I do that stuff all the time. What's the big deal?" Because I had kept their work so private, and not made a big deal about it, Jason just couldn't figure it out. All I said was, "Sometimes adults do silly things like that." And that was it; he did not ask any more questions. I don't want my boys to think they are any different from the rest of their classmates because of their work. Nicholas was confronted with a similar situation when he first appeared locally in a commercial for PlayWorld airing on the Fox Network. This time the kids were simply more curious than anything else because they saw someone they knew on television while they were eating their breakfast before school. Ah, the innocence of children—I love it!

Being involved in this industry does bring added attention to your family if their work is seen locally. I noticed that when my children reached school age, no matter how private I had kept their involvement in the past, it was now out of my hands to a certain degree. That comes with the territory and is something one must accept while participating in this field.

Growing up is a challenge no matter where we live or what our kids are involved in, whether the activities are sports, music, theater, or whatever. There is no real difference between trying out for a school soccer team or auditioning for a commercial. Some teams they will make and some they will not. It is our job as parents to support our children in all that they do; and remind them, if they ever have doubts about themselves, that it's not winning the game or the audition that counts, but that journey down the road that makes them feel like a winner, no matter what the end result may be. Praise and love at any age goes a long way.

Obtaining Copies of Your Children's Work

After Jason had completed filming his first commercial, how would I be able to see it? It was going to air in Iowa! This is how I have gone about obtaining Jason's and Nicholas' work. Most producers and advertising agencies do not want to be bothered by parents who want copies of their kids' work. Providing copies could end up being a full-time job in itself. I have been very fortunate to obtain copies of almost all the work that my boys have done, by being very casual, careful, and polite about it.

By the end of a shoot, I can usually tell who is running things. It is hard to find the opportunity to talk to these people without others being around, so I take one step at a time. I approach the person in charge when he or she is not surrounded by the other talent and ask for a business card. The person in charge is either from the production company or the advertising company; both may have access to copies. If, after receiving their business card, I can continue the conversation, I ask if I can contact them in a couple of weeks to obtain a copy of the video, print, or whatever medium the job was for. If it is a video tape copy, I send a blank tape with a self-addressed stamped manila padded envelope, to make it as easy as possible for them to comply with my request. Or just bring it with me and give it to the person in charge, if they will accept it. For print work, I don't know what type or size of print they will send me, so I do not send an envelope unless requested.

I have received all different kinds of copies. One advertising agency actually sent me a copy of the print that Jason did for Sears clothes line, a 20 x 20 blow-up on a foam-backed board. It was wonderful! And some have sent me the color copy negative to allow me to make whatever size I needed. Jason received a job to be one of the first group of kids to advertise a new line of vitamins. The advertising company was wonderful and sent me copies of the ad laminated in placemat form. We were told at the shoot that those first kids, if everything worked out as planned, would likely be appearing in more of the vitiamin ads and commercials. Unfortunately, the whole project was canceled shortly thereafter. I cannot say exactly what happened; however, the company for which the advertisement was being made had just made a business deal with another company. Vitamins with characters from that other company were soon on the market.

I have been very fortunate to receive what I have. I think my success depends on a combination of the approach, the timing and the personality of the individual I am dealing with. It is important, though, to respect and accept the individual's response if it is negative. The way I look at it, I can't go wrong by just asking.

Promoting *Along* with the Talent Agency

My mind hardly stops thinking of ways to gain more knowledge about this industry and find more ways to promote my boys, in addition to being registered with the agencies.

Once you have signed with a talent agency, you should keep the agency updated with current photos and resumes, as you already should know from reading the previous chapters. A lack of photos probably means no audition calls. Reading newsletters or industry publications could help you. BOXOFFICE Magazine has much information on the who, what and where of the movie industry's upcoming projects before scripts are even written. Consider subscribing if that is an area you wish to pursue once you have become registered and are comfortable with what you are doing. Also available is my quarterly newsletter of updated information (see page 135, for information on how to subscribe).

Self-promoting by contacting casting agencies yourself is permissible as long as you obey the rules. A casting agency, as I understand it, is the inside connection which is usually hired by either the production company or the advertising agency. The casting agent in turn contacts the talent agency (with which we are registered) and works directly with the talent agency staff, who will notify the talent (the actors or models) and set up audition times for an upcoming project. Please understand the difference between casting and talent agencies and don't confuse them. I have always been told and have read many times, that talent never calls a casting agent. Respect their rules! You may send in composites and a resume telling them which talent agency you are registered with, but that is it. I cannot stress this enough. Your talent agency works closely with the casting agency, and, if the latter has received your composites or snapshots, either from the talent agency you are registered with or from you, and the casting agent wants to see your child in on a audition, he or she will contact your talent agency.

One time I spoke on the phone with a casting agency employee, who had called _me_ following an audition, and after our talent agency had closed. Jason received the the job, which was the next day. Time was of the essence, so a casting staff member called directly to give me the needed information. The only other time I spoke to someone at a casting agency was when I called the agency regarding an audition call that had been cancelled. I was put in my place, though, not only by the casting people but also by the talent agency that had sent us to the audition. I realized that when we are told not to call the casting people, they mean it! Follow the rules and be courteous.

Casting Information

In some of the casting information that follows, you may see comments from the casting agencies. Pay close attention to those notes and follow the instructions precisely. I have compiled a useful list of all sorts of casting information, with help from The CD Directory, a comprehensive guide to casting directors, and The Ross Reports. I have also included the address of the Casting Society of America (see Bibliography, at the back of the book), which will allow you to write to obtain the current list of casting agencies listed with the Society. When you do write to your local SAG office for their current talent agent list, you can ask them to send you any addresses of casting agencies and directors as well. Some will send them and some won't. It doesn't hurt to ask.

I have been granted permission to reprint a few pages of some of key publications. The names and addresses in these books are just what one needs to contact important people in the industry in addition to the talent agencies. However, you should be registered with a talent agency first. Included, are names of people who cast for such great television shows as *Home Improvement, Lois and Clark: The New Adventures of Superman,* etc. I have found that The Ross Reports and The CD Directory complement each other. By reading The Ross Reports and finding the television show you want to send a composite to, you will find the appropriate casting person's name listed. Now look in The CD Directory alphabetical listing and find the address. Once again, the same rule applies—no phone calls. You can subscribe to these publications for the most up-to-date information about each show.

TV PRO-LOG DIGEST
TELEVISION PROGRAMS AND PRODUCTION NEWS

Those folks who brought us **Dynasty**, Richard and Esther Shapiro, are working on a two-hour pilot for ABC. The network has ordered the pilot and six additional scripts, in case the pilot is a success. The project will feature several families and an undercurrent of police investigation. The Shapiros will executive produce through their Shapiro Entertainment, in association with All American TV, the distributors of the syndicated hit **Baywatch**. This is the first network production for All American. John Whelpley will write and produce the pilot, which will be directed by Tim Hunter. No, not me - the other Tim Hunter who directed the **Beverly Hills, 90210** pilot, episodes of **Twin Peaks,** and the feature films **Tex** and **The River's Edge**..............Ah, this is interesting. For this season, ABC ordered 19 episodes of **All-American Girl** from Sandollar TV, Heartfelt Productions (Gary Jacobs) and Touchstone TV Eighteen of the episodes will be business as usual. But, the nineteenth episode will, in essence, be a pilot for a new show featuring series star Margaret Cho and Amy Hill, who play's Cho's grandmother on **All-American Girl**. So next year, ABC will have the option of ordering a second season of **All-American Girl** or the new show starring Margaret Cho. Or neither. It has yet to be determined whether the new pilot will be broadcast this spring or merely used as a template for the possible reworking of the existing series..............There is no escape. Next season, ABC will air an animated series based on the film **Dumb and Dumber.** Yes folks, Hanna-Barbera and New Line Television are animating the inept duo, Harry and Lloyd. And, you can bet those three-inch figurines will be stores shortly after the premiere of the series. And you thought you were afraid for your child's future now..............ABC News will open a new computerized tape and film historical footage library in April that will feature archival stock footage from both ABC News and the film and video libraries of Worldwide Television News (WTN). The library of WTN represents the largest group of news archives in the world. The new facility, dubbed ABC News Videosource, will include all major news events covered by ABC News since 1963, as well as extensive outtakes shot at the same time, but never seen before. The material will be easily accessed via a

SPECIAL TALENT GROUPS (Not Unions)

ALL-TAME ANIMALS (Animals Only)   (212) 245-6740
  457 West 57th Street
  New York, New York 10019
    Contact: Barbara Weir
ANTELOPE TO ZEBRA AGENCY (Animals Only) (201) 729-3442
  19 Indian Trail, Sparta, New Jersey 07871
    Contact: Eddy Lester (Contact by mail first)
AUSTRALIAN NEW ZEALAND ARTISTS ALLIANCE
  228 West 71st Street, # 2F   (212) 229-7864
  New York, New York 10023
    Contact: John Roddick
CASTING SOCIETY OF AMERICA   (212) 333-4552
  311 West 43rd Street
  New York, New York 10036

SPECIAL TALENT GROUP (Not Union) (Cont'd)

HISPANIC ORGANIZATION OF LATIN ACTORS (HOLA)
  250 West 65th Street, New York 10023-6403 (212) 595-8286
LEAGUE OF INDEPENDENT STUNTPLAYERS (212) 777-7021
  P.O. Box 19C, Madison Square Station
  New York, New York 10159
    Contact: David Copeland
**NATIONAL ASSOCIATION OF TALENT
REPRESENTATIVES (NATR)**   (212) 752-4968
  Address to be announced
    Contact: Lee Buckler
NATIONAL CONFERENCE OF PERSONAL MANAGERS
  1650 Broadway, Suite 705, New York 10019 (212) 265-3366
    Contact: Joseph Rapp.
ON LOCATION EDUCATION   (212) 222-2302
  (Certified Teachers for Television, Film, and Theatre)
  175 West 92nd Street, Suite 1D, New York 10025
    Contact: Alan Simon, Director
TUTORING FOR CHILDREN LTD. (Certified Teachers for
  Television, Film and Theatre)   (212) 557-7890
  245 East 40th Street, # 31C, New York 10016
    Contact: Shelley Zacharia

NEW YORK PRODUCERS OF TV COMMERCIALS

NOTE: This list of New York producers of television commercials includes many who are signatories of agreements with Screen Actors Guild (*) or American Federation of Television and Radio Artists (+). Others are contract or independent producers who work with agencies or advertisers who are signatories of the union agreements. Some producers who specialize in animation (**A**) are also listed. (**Y**) indicates those producers that accept pictures and resumes for in-house casting files.

AKERS/ROBINS/FERNBACH   (212) 879-8787
  510 East 74th Street, New York 10021
ARTISTS COMPANY / A & R GROUP (Y) (212) 679-7199
  38 West 21st Street, New York 10010
GENNARO ANDREOZZI INC.   (212) 477-4200
  118 East 25th Street, New York 10010
ELBERT BUDON, INC (*)   (212) 673-0334
  32 West 10th Street, New York 10011
CROSSROADS FILMS   (212) 647-1300
  136 West 21st Street, 5th Floor, New York 10011

ROSS REPORTS

NETWORK PRIMETIME PROGRAMS
1994-95 SEASON

Basic program listings for all network primetime programs, except movies (made for television and theatrical), or documentary or public affairs series. Times listed are current New York Time. Studios are listed with full addresses on the page preceding this one. Production and other credits are added to listings as they become available or are changed.

*indicates completely new listing
Vertical black line indicates deletion or change in listing or information since previous issue

ABC

FAMILY MATTERS   Comedy
Fridays, 8-8:30pm - Film   (Sixth Season)
JoMarie Payton Noble, Reginald VelJohnson, Rosetta LeNoire, Darius McCrary, Kellie Shanygne Williams, Jaleel White, Michele Thomas, Shawn Harrison & Bryton McClure star.
PKGR: Bickley-Warren Productions with Miller/Boyett Productions and Warner Bros. TV at Warner Bros. Studios. EXEC PRODS: Thomas L. Miller & Robert L. Boyett (developers), William Bickley & Michael Warren (creators), David W. Duclon. SUPERV PRODS: Fred Fox, Jr., Jim Geoghan. PRODS: Kelly Sandefur, Stephen Langford, Sara V. Finney & Vida Spears. CO-PROD: Rebecca Misra. CONSULT: Gary Menteer. CASTING: Barbara Miller and Geraldine Leder.

FULL HOUSE   Comedy
Tuesdays, 8-8:30pm - Tape   (Eighth Season)
John Stamos, Bob Saget, Dave Coulier, Candace Cameron, Jodie Sweetin, Mary-Kate and Ashley Olsen, Lori Loughlin, Blake & Dylan Twomy-Wilhoit, Andrea Barber star.
PKGR: Jeff Franklin Prods/Miller-Boyett Prods/Warner Bros. TV at Warner Bros. Studios. EXEC PRODS: Thomas L. Miller & Robert L. Boyett, Jeff Franklin, Marc Warren & Dennis Rinsler. CO-EXEC PRODS: Don Van Atta, Ellen Guylas. SUPERV PROD: Tom Amundsen. PRODS: James O'Keefe, Bonnie Bogard Maier, Greg Fields, Jamie & Chuck Tatham. COORD PROD: Miles Kristman. EXEC STORY EDS: Adam I. Lapidus, Carolyn Omine. CREATOR: Jeff Franklin. CASTING: Barbara Miller and Joanne Koehler.

GRACE UNDER FIRE   Comedy
Tuesdays, 9:30-10pm - Film   (Second Season)
Brett Butler, Dave Thomas, Julie White, Casey Sander, Jon Paul Steuer, Kaitlin Cullum, Dylan & Cole Sprouse star.
PKGR: Carsey-Werner Company at CBS Studio Center. EXEC PRODS: Marcy Carsey, Tom Werner, Caryn Mandabach, Marc Flanagan. CO-EXEC PROD: Jeff Abugov. SUPERV PRODS: Bob Dolan Smith, Kathy Ann Stumpe. PRODS: Joanne Curley Kerner, J.J. Wall. CO-PRODS: Hollis Rich, Brenda Hanes-Berg, Bill Masters. EXEC STORY ED: Paul Raley. EXEC CONSULT: Brett Butler. CREATIVE CONSULTS: Karen Hall, Chuck Lorre (creator). CASTING: Liberman/Hirschfeld.

ROSS REPORTS

HOME IMPROVEMENT   Comedy
Tuesdays, 9-9:30pm - Tape   (Fourth Season)
   Starring Tim Allen, Patricia Richardson, Jonathan Taylor
   Thomas, Taran Noah Smith, Zachery Ty Bryan, Earl Hindman
   & Richard Karn.
PKGR: Wind Dancer Prods, Inc./Touchstone TV at Disney Studios.
EXEC PRODS: Elliot Shoenman & Bob Bendetson, Bruce Ferber.
EXEC PRODS & CREATORS: Matt Williams, Carmen Finestra,
David McFadzean. PRODS: Andy Cadiff, Frank McKemy, Howard J.
Morris. CO-PRODS: Rosalind Moore & Jim Praytor. CONSULT
PRODS: Gayle S. Maffeo, Billy Riback. EXEC CONSULT: Tim
Allen. CREATIVE CONSULTS: Marley Sims, Lloyd Garver.
CASTING: Deborah Barylski. ✱

LOIS & CLARK:
THE NEW ADVENTURES OF SUPERMAN   Action-Adventures
Sundays, 8-9pm - Film   (Second Season)
   Dean Cain, Teri Hatcher, Lane Smith, Justin Whalin, K Callan &
   Eddie Jones star.
PKGR: December 3rd Prods/Warner Bros. TV. EXEC PROD:
Robert Singer. CO-EXEC PROD: James Crocker. SUPERV PRODS:
Tony Blake & Paul Jackson, Randall Zisk. CO-PRODS: Philip J.
Sgriccia, John McNamara, Jim Michaels. EXEC CONSULT:
Deborah Joy LeVine (creator). CREATIVE CONSULT: Kathy
McCormick. CASTING: Barbara Miller, Ellie Kanner.

THE MARSHAL   Drama
Saturdays, 10-11pm - Film   (First Season)
   Jeff Fahey stars as U.S. Marshal Winston MacBride, searching
   for fugutives from justice.
PKGR: Buffalo Wallet Prods/Western Sandblast/Paramount TV.
EXEC PRODS: Daniel Pyne, John Mankiewicz, Aaron Lipstadt, Don
Johnson. PRODS: Gareth Davies, Terry Curtis Fox, Hans Tobeason.
CO-PROD: Diane Sillan. CREATORS: John Mankiewicz & Daniel
Pyne. CASTING: Pagano/Manwiller (LA); Michelle Allen (Canada)

NYPD BLUE   Police Dramas
Tuesdays, 10-11pm - Film   (Second Season)
   Starring Jimmy Smits, Dennis Franz, James McDaniel, Nicholas
   Turturro, Sharon Lawrence, Gordon Clapp, Gail O'Grady.
PKGR: Steven Bochco Prods/Twentieth Television at 20th Century-
Fox Studios. EXEC PRODS: Steven Bochco & David Milch (crea-
tors). CO-EXEC PRODS: Charles H. Eglee & Channing Gibson,
Walon Green. SUPERV PROD: Michael M. Robin. PROD: Ted
Mann. CO-PRODS: Burton Armus, Gardner Stern, Steven DePaul.
COORD PROD: Robert J. Doherty. CONSULT PROD: Bill Clark.
CASTING: Junie Lowry-Johnson (LA); Alexa Fogel (NY) (See p. 34);
Byron Crystal (NY extras). (See p. 4)

ROSS REPORTS

To find Deborah Barylski casting director of Home Improvements see CD Diectory Alphabetical Listing

ALPHABETICAL LISTING

— A —

RACHEL ABROMS (Rachel Abroms Casting) CSA 213-871-2107
2486 Cheremoya Ave. (Los Angeles) 90068

CECILY ADAMS (Independent) 818-569-7356

MERCEDES ALBERTI-PENNEY (Independent)
2144 Rockledge Road (Los Angeles) 90068

JULIE ALTER (Independent) CSA 213-463-1925
6565 Sunset Blvd., #306 (Los Angeles) 90028

DONNA ANDERSON (Independent) CSA 213-463-1925
CSA, 6565 Sunset Blvd., #306 (Los Angeles) 90028

MEI LING ANDREEN (New Star Casting) 818-785-3305
P.O. Box 2626 (Beverly Hills) 90213

DEBORAH AQUILA (Paramount Studios) CSA 213-956-5444
VP of Casting, Motion Pictures, Paramount Studios, 5555 Melrose Ave., Bob Hope Bldg., #200 (LA) 90028

MAUREEN ARATA (Maureen Arata Casting) CSA 818-777-4410
Universal Studios, 100 Universal City Plaza, Bldg. 506, #A104 (Universal City) 91608

MARY GAIL ARTZ (Artz/Cohen Casting) 213-463-3831
6525 Sunset Blvd., Garden Suite 11 (Los Angeles) 90028

JEANNE ASHBY (Barbara Remsen & Associates) 213-464-7968
Raleigh Studios, 650 N. Bronson Ave., #124 (Los Angeles) 90004

JULIE ASHTON (Mike Fenton & Associates) 818-501-0177
14724 Ventura Blvd., #510 (Sherman Oaks) 91403

NINA AXELROD (Independent) 303-963-0353
Rocky Mountain Talent, P.O. Box 558 (Snowmass) 81654

SIMON AYER (Hymson/Ayer Casting) CSA 818-972-0303
Glen Larson Productions, 3400 Riverside Drive, 3rd Floor (Burbank) 91505

— B —

RISE BARISH (Independent-Commercials) CCDA 310-276-0655
143 S. Spalding Drive (Beverly Hills) 90212

CAROL BARLOW (Prime Casting-Commercials) 213-962-0377
7060 Hollywood Blvd., #1025 (Los Angeles) 90028

ANTHONY BARNAO (Independent) 213-993-5662
846 N. Cahuenga Blvd., Bldg. A, #105 (Los Angeles) 90038

DEBORAH BARYLSKI (Deborah Barylski Casting) CSA 818-560-2896
The Walt Disney Studios, 500 S. Buena Vista St., Trailer T31 (Burbank) 91521

PARAMOUNT STUDIOS. .... 956-5000 .... 5555 Melrose Avenue (L.A.) 90038
    Helen Mossler .... 956-5578 (VP of Talent)
    Deborah Aquila .... 956-5444 (VP of Casting, Motion Pictures)
    Jane Shannon .... 956-5480 (Manager of Casting, Motion Pictures)

    Independents At Paramount
  * Pamela Basker 956-3813
  * Nan Dutton 956-8183
    Jeff Greenberg 956-4886
    Cara Coslow
    Sheila Guthrie
    Tory Herald 956-4141
  * Junie Lowry-Johnson 956-4856
    Ron Surma
    Jeff Oshen 956-4850
    Sharon Soble
    Richard Pagano 956-4141
    Sharon Bialy
    Susan Booker
    Allison Kohler
    Debi Manwiller
    Gretchen Rennell 956-4288

TELEVISION CENTER. .... 464-6638 .... 6311 Romaine St. (L.A.) 90038

    Independents At Television Center
    Kathleen Letterie 962-5575
    Heidi Levitt 467-7400
    Rick Montgomery 461-3399
    Dan Parada
    Julie Mossberg 469-2804

INDEPENDENTS *Organized by zip code*
    Dennis Gallegos .... 469-3577 .... 611 N. Larchmont Blvd., 1st Floor (L.A.) 90004
    Ann Wilkinson
  * Meg Liberman .... 346-8225 .... Hewitt Studios, 130 S. Hewitt St. (L.A.) 90012
  * Irene Cagen
    Janet Cunningham .... 461-2000 .... 5205 Hollywood Blvd., #211 (L.A.) 90027
    Bob Morones .... 953-5657 .... KCET, 4401 Sunset Blvd. (L.A.) 90027
    Stephen Snyder .... 465-4241 .... 1801 N. Kingsley Dr., #202 (L.A.) 90027
    James Pantone .... 953-1200 .... 1662 Hillhurst Ave. (L.A.) 90027
    Lisa Pantone
    Leslee Dennis .... 462-4705 .... 1680 N. Vine St., #1200 (L.A.) 90028
    Deborah Kurtz .... 461-3800 .... 1600 N. Highland Ave., #4 (L.A.) 90028
    Megan McConnell .... 463-8655 .... 7060 Hollywood Blvd., #604 (L.A.) 90028
    Gary Oberst .... 463-7872 .... 1260 N. Wilcox, #9 (L.A.) 90028
    Renee Rousselot .... 463-8655 .... 7060 Hollywood Blvd., #604 (L.A.) 90028
    Melanie Sherwood .... 462-6817 .... 6305 Yucca St., #600 (L.A.) 90028
    Linda Francis .... 467-3838 .... Planet Productions, 1645 N. Vine St., #706 (L.A.) 90028
    Yumi Takada .... 962-3025 .... 1400 N. Orange Dr. (L.A.) 90028
    Risa Bramon Garcia .... 469-7303 .... 6404 Hollywood Blvd., #309 (L.A.) 90028
    Mary Vernieu
    Mary Gail Artz .... 463-3831 .... 6525 Sunset Blvd., Garden Suite 11 (L.A.) 90028
    Barbara Cohen
    Jack Jones .... 464-9216 .... 5858 Hollywood Blvd., #220 (L.A.) 90028
    Carol Barlow .... 962-0377 .... 7060 Hollywood Blvd., #1025 (L.A.) 90028
    Shancy Pierce .... 469-8233 .... 6305 Yucca St., #211 (L.A.) 90028
    Loree Booth .... 464-2788 .... 6521 Homewood Ave. (L.A.) 90028
    Leland Williams
  * Ira Belgrade .... 938-3800 .... 5850-E W. 3rd St.,(L.A.) 90036
    Michael Lien .... 937-0411 .... 7461 Beverly Blvd., #203 (L.A.) 90036
    Myrna Meth .... 653-8119 .... 442 1/2 N. Ogden Dr. (L.A.) 90036
    Ross Brown .... 938-2575 .... 7319 Beverly Blvd., #10 (L.A.) 90036
    Mary West

CD DIRECTORY

BREAKDOWN SERVICES'
CASTING DIRECTOR ASSIGNMENTS FOR THE 1994/1995 SEASON
Please note: This list was compiled using all currently available information, which may change at any time.

TITLE	CASTING DIRECTOR	PRODUCTION COMPANY	NETWORK
ALL AMERICAN GIRL	NIKKI VALKO	DISNEY	ABC
ALL MY CHILDREN	JUDY WILSON - NY	ABC PRODUCTIONS	ABC
AMERICA'S MOST WANTED	VARIOUS	STF/FOX	FOX
ANOTHER WORLD	JOHNSON/MARX - NY		
	RICK MILLIKAN - LA	PROCTER & GAMBLE	NBC
AS THE WORLD TURNS	VINCE LIEBHART - NY	PROCTER & GAMBLE	CBS
BABYLON 5	SLATER/BROOKSBANK	RATTLESNAKE/WARNER	SYN
BAYWATCH	GLICKSMAN/ORENSTEIN	BAYWATCH PRODUCTIONS	SYN
BEVERLY HILLS, 90210	DIANNE YOUNG	AARON SPELLING	FOX
BLOSSOM	MEYER/ROBERTS	WITT/THOMAS/HARRIS	NBC
BLUE SKIES	DAVA WAITE	UNIVERSAL	ABC
BOLD & THE BEAUTIFUL	CHRISTY DOOLEY	BELL/PHILLIPS	CBS
BOY MEETS WORLD	SALLY STINER	DISNEY	ABC
THE BOYS ARE BACK	NAN DUTTON	ABC PRODUCTIONS	CBS
BROTHER TO BROTHER	GERALDINE LEDER	WARNER BROS. TV	SYN
BURKE'S LAW	DENISE CHAMIAN	AARON SPELLING	CBS
CALIFORNIA DREAMS	ROBIN LIPPIN	NBC PRODUCTIONS	NBC
CARLIN	MARK SAKS	WARNER BROS. TV	FOX
CHICAGO HOPE	STEVEN JACOBS	TWENTIETH TV	CBS
CHRISTY	PENNY ELLERS		
	JO DOSTER - TENNESSEE	FAMILY	CBS
COACH	DAVA WAITE	UNIVERSAL	ABC
THE COMMISH	BRAD WARSHAW		
	SUZANNE MCLELLAN - VANCOUVER	STEPHEN J. CANNELL	ABC
THE COSBY MYSTERIES	HUGHES/MOSS - NY	NBC/COLUMBIA	NBC
COSMIC SLOP	EILEEN MACK KNIGHT	HUDLIN BROTHERS	HBO
DADDY'S GIRLS	JULIE MOSSBERG	WITT/THOMAS	CBS
DAVE'S WORLD	LISA MIONIE	CBS/FRED BARRON	CBS
DAYS OF OUR LIVES	FRAN BASCOM	COLUMBIA PICTURES TV	NBC
DIAGNOSIS MURDER	MAUREEN ARATA	VIACOM	CBS
DOUBLE RUSH	ANDREA COHEN	SHUKOVSKY/ENGLISH	CBS
DR. QUINN, MEDICINE WOMAN	ALAN HOCHBERG	CBS ENTERTAINMENT	CBS
DREAM ON	TRACY LILIENFIELD	MEKLIS	HBO
DUE SOUTH	LISA LONDON		
	CLAIRE WALKER - TORONTO	ALLIANCE	CBS
EARTH II	MEGAN BRANMAN	AMBLIN/UNIVERSAL	NBC
ELLEN	TAMMY BILLIK	BLACK/MARLENS	ABC
EMPTY NEST	CAMI PATTON	WITT/THOMAS	NBC
ENCOUNTERS	PATRICK RUSH	BERKELEY GROUP	FOX
ER	JOHN LEVEY	AMBLIN/WARNER BROS. TV	NBC
FAMILY MATTERS	GERALDINE LEDER	WARNER BROS. TV	ABC
FIVE MRS. BUCHANANS	ALLISON JONES	TWENTIETH TV	CBS
FORTUNE HUNTER	SLATER/BROOKSBANK		
	MEL JOHNSON - ORLANDO	COLUMBIA PICTURES TV	FOX
FRASIER	JEFF GREENBERG	PARAMOUNT	NBC
FRESH PRINCE OF BEL AIR	LISA MILLER	NBC/QUINCY JONES	NBC
FRIENDS	ELLIE KANNER	WARNER BROS. TV	NBC
FUDGE	MEGAN FOLEY	AMBLIN	ABC
FULL HOUSE	JOANNE KOEHLER	WARNER BROS. TV	ABC
GENERAL HOSPITAL	MARK TESCHNER	ABC PRODUCTIONS	ABC
GET SMART	SALLY STINER	HBO INDEPENDENT	FOX
GRACE UNDER FIRE	LIBERMAN/HIRSCHFELD	CARSEY/WERNER	ABC
GREAT DEFENDER	TONY SEPULVEDA	WARNER BROS. TV	FOX
GUIDING LIGHT	BETTY REA - NY	PROCTER & GAMBLE	CBS
HANGIN' WITH MR. COOPER	DEEDEE BRADLEY	WARNER BROS. TV	ABC
HARDBALL	BRIAN CHAVANNE	DISNEY	FOX
HARLEQUIN ROMANCES	NAN DUTTON		
	BUCHAN/TAIT - TORONTO	ALLIANCE	CBS
HAWKEYE	LUCY CAVALLO		
	CAROL KELSAY - VANCOUVER	STEPHEN J. CANNELL	SYN

CD DIRECTORY

TITLE	CASTING DIRECTOR	PRODUCTION COMPANY	NETWORK
HEARTS AFIRE	FRAN BASCOM	COLUMBIA/MOZARK/ADAM	CBS
HEAVEN HELP US	ULRICH/DAWSON	AARON SPELLING	SYN
HEAVENS TO BETSY	BUCK/EDELMAN	SANDDOLLAR	CBS
HIDDEN WORLD OF ALEX MACK	JOEY PAUL	LYNCH ENTERTAINMENT	NICK
HIGHLANDER	PAMELA BASKER		
	TRISH ROBINSON - VANCOUVER	RYSHER/GAUMONT/FILMLINE	SYN
HOME IMPROVEMENT	DEBORAH BARYLSKI	WIND DANCER/DISNEY	ABC
HOMICIDE	LOU DIGIAIMO - NEW YORK	BALTIMORE PICTURES	NBC
HOTEL MALIBU	DENISE CHAMIAN	LATHAM/LECHOWICK	CBS
HOUSE OF BUGGIN'	MARCIA SHULMAN	HBO INDEPENDENT	FOX
IN THE HEAT OF THE NIGHT	JAN GLASER	MGM/UA	CBS
KUNG FU	SUSAN FORREST	WARNER BROS. TV	SYN
JOHN LARROQUETTE SHOW	KATHLEEN LETTERIE	WITT/THOMAS	NBC
LARRY SANDERS SHOW	LIBERMAN/HIRSCHFELD	BRILLSTEIN/GREY	HBO
LAW & ORDER	KRESSEL/RYAN - NY	UNIVERSAL	NBC
LIVING SINGLE	GERALDINE LEDER	WARNER BROS. TV	FOX
LOIS AND CLARK	ELLIE KANNER	WARNER BROS. TV	ABC
LONESOME DOVE	LESLIE SWAN	CANADIAN DOVE, INC.	SYN
LOVE AND WAR	ANDREA COHEN	SHUKOVSKY/ENGLISH	CBS
LOVE LINE	FRANCIS/MONAHAN	MAGIC HOUR	HBO/
CINEMAX			
LOVE STREET	LAURA FRANCIS	ENCOUNTER FILMS	SHOWTIME
LOVING	JULIE MADISON - NY		
	NICK WILKINSON - LA	ABC PRODUCTIONS	ABC
MAD ABOUT YOU	VASH/NATHAN	TRISTAR	NBC
MADISON	TRISH ROBINSON - VANCOUVER	FOREFRONT	GLOBAL
MADMAN OF THE PEOPLE	LIBERMAN/HIRSCHFELD/KATCHER	AARON SPELLING	NBC
M.A.N.T.I.S.	ELLEN LUBIN SANITSKY		
	STUART AIKINS - VANCOUVER	UNIVERSAL	FOX
MARRIED, WITH CHILDREN	VICKIE ROSENBERG	COLUMBIA PICTURES TV	FOX
THE MARSHALL	PAGANO/BIALY/MANWILLER/HERALD		
	MICHELLE ALLEN - VANCOUVER	PARAMOUNT	ABC
MARTIN	KIM WILLIAMS	HBO INDEPENDENT	FOX
MARTIN SHORT SHOW	LIBERMAN/HIRSCHFELD	NBC PRODUCTIONS	NBC
MATLOCK	ULRICH/DAWSON/KRITZER	VIACOM	ABC
MCKENNA	RAY/HUZZAR	ABC PRODUCTIONS	ABC
ME & THE BOYS	MONICA SWANN	ABC PRODUCTIONS/MYER	ABC
MEDICINE BALL	TED HANN	LAKESIDE	FOX
MELROSE PLACE	DEBRA RUBINSTEIN	AARON SPELLING	FOX
MODELS, INC.	PENNY ELLERS	AARON SPELLING	FOX
THE MOMMIES	JEFF OSHEN	PARAMOUNT	NBC
MUDDLING THROUGH	LAPADURA/HART	CBS/COLUMBIA PICTURES TV	CBS
MURDER SHE WROTE	RON STEPHENSON	UNIVERSAL	CBS
MURPHY BROWN	ANDREA COHEN	WARNER BROS. TV	CBS
MY BROTHER & ME	MICHAEL KOEGEL		
	JENNIFER VAN DER MOLEN - ORLANDO	NICKELODEON	NICK
MY SO-CALLED LIFE	JEFF GREENBERG	ABC PRODUCTIONS	ABC
MYSTERIOUS ISLAND	WINTHROP/KAPLAN		
	SUSAN FORREST - NEW ZEALAND	ATLANTIS	SYN
THE NANNY	APRIL WEBSTER	STERNIN & FRASER/TRISTAR	CBS
NEW YORK UNDERCOVER	LYNN KRESSEL - NY	UNIVERSAL	FOX
NORTHERN EXPOSURE	MEGAN BRANMAN		
	DIXON/WALKER - SEATTLE	PIPELINE	CBS
NORTHWOOD	SID KOZAK - VANCOUVER	OMNI	CBC
NYPD BLUE	SUSAN BLUESTEIN	BOCHCO	ABC
THE ODYSSEY	SID KOZAK - VANCOUVER	WATERSTREET PICTURES	CBC
THE OFFICE	CAMI PATTON	WITT/THOMAS	CBS
ONE LIFE TO LIVE	ELLEN NOVACK - NY	ABC PRODUCTIONS	ABC
ONE WEST WAIKIKI	HYMSON/AYER	LARSON/RYSHER	CBS
ON OUR OWN	TONY SEPULVEDA	WARNER BROS. TV	ABC
PARTY OF FIVE	LIBERMAN/HIRSCHFELD/RUSH	COLUMBIA PICTURES TV	FOX
PERRY MASON	ULRICH/DAWSON/KRITZER	VIACOM	NBC
PICKET FENCES	PAGANO/BIALY/MANWILLER	TWENTIETH TV	CBS
POINTMAN	DEEDEE BRADLEY	POINTMAN	SYN
POWER RANGERS	KATY WALLIN	MMPR	SYN
PUZZLEWORKS	BOB MORONES	KCET	PBS

Finding the Right Balance Between Opportunity and Family

The door is wide open for you and for me, but it really depends on how much work we want for our children. The more persistent one is, the more it could pay off, but not without risking our children's and our own normal way of life. How much one wants to self-promote is a decision that should be thought out completely. If I were to contact one of the network show casting directors by sending in Jason's and Nicholas' composites with their resumes and a cover letter, would I be prepared to accept a job offer which might take us away from our home, our family, and the boys' school now that they are older, or which may require that we relocate as did Zachery Bryan's (from the famous tool sitcom) family? Will our children have a hard time fitting back into a normal way of life after the all the fuss is over on the movie set? Chapter 8, Sharing Thoughts of Others Growing Up in the Industry, contains excerpts from interviews with young actors who discuss how acting has affected their personal lives.

Nicholas auditioned for the part of one of Tom Arnold's son's neighborhood friends, then was called back on a second audition for Tom Arnold's son, Jack, Jr., instead. This was for a movie called "Graceland," which never made it to the big screen. The movie was also to star Arnold's wife at that time, Roseanne Barr. The director, Bill Bixby, was coming in from L. A. for that audition. Unexpectly things were moving so fast. I was so excited—we were getting up to the big league now. Then, at the last minute, everything was called off with no explanation. We had to figure it all out ourselves based on what we read in the papers.

You know how they say things happen for a reason? The cancellation of that movie gave me a chance to think about a situation that I had not thought about carefully enough before. The movie was going to be filmed on location in Iowa. If Nicholas had received the role, we would have had to stay in Iowa for a minimum of three weeks. Now, was this what I really wanted? Nicholas and I away from my older son Jason and Randy, my husband, and our family business? The boys and I enjoy being in this field, and Dad doesn't mind it either because it does not control our regular lives. Landing a part in a movie roll or a series offer could make things difficult. Try to consider all factors when you are self-promoting, as well as what you audition through the agency. Don't audition for something you

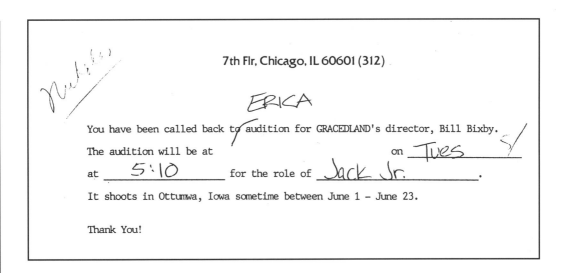

may not be able to accept. Sort out in your own mind; do you want an eight-million dollar son like the main actor in "Home Alone," who went trick or treating for the first time at age thirteen? Or will doing commercials, industrial videos and print work, that keeps you and your child closer to home, be enough? I have come to realize that I prefer the latter at this point in our lives.

Managing Your Children's Income

Jason and Nicholas have not made millions, but they certainly have more money put away than a lot of kids their age. For children, that is one of the benefits of the business. As their parents, it is our job to see that the money they make is put away for their future. Saving bonds, savings accounts, mutual funds, and stocks all bear my sons' names, and the boys are only 10 and 12. Oh, sure, I could reimburse myself for the travel expenses, their photos, and clothes, but I don't. This is my choice. Just like in sports, I have to bring them to and from their games, purchase their clothes, and team photos anyway. But, the big difference between sports and modeling is that they get paid for participating in the modeling field when they received the job. Why not just put whatever they make away? I'm sure both boys' will appreciate it later on. I oftened wondered how many parents actually do save their kids money for the future? Unless you live in certain areas, that have a statue regulating how a minors earnings are put aside, the parent is free to do whatever they please regarding handling a minors earnings. So we must do it wisely. This is an area one must search out professionals in the legal and investment fields, for advise.

Final Anecdotes: Tales of Terror and Triumph!

People encounter all types of situations, in life and the modeling field is no exception. I have had the joy of watching baby Jason crawl his way into the hearts of the people in Iowa for the healthcare company with his double dimpled smile. He has left his image in print advertisements for magazines and newspapers, in commercials, and in industrial videos for big-name companies such as McDonald's, Amway, and Whirlpool, to name a few. And Nicholas, in spite of him missing his front tooth at age 3, that kept his auditioning to a minimum, still he has been able to visit his classmates during their breakfast or afternoon snack whenever his commercial for "PlayWorld" appeared on their televisions.

On many of these auditions and jobs we were treated with professionalism and enjoyed very nice settings. We have been pampered and fussed over; Have been photograghed at very elaborate homes and modern high rise studios that seemed to have come right out of a magazine. These experiences make this business so intriguing.

However, we have run into the dark side of this business as well. Even top New York agencies will put aside consideration for the comfort of the talent and close their eyes to the environment in which the shoot takes place. Some advertising companies have only one thing in mind - the end result, what they want to portray in the final shot. If the job I am about to describe had been one of our first, we probably would not have stayed in this business. But it was, I am happy to say, the only situation of this kind we encountered.

When Nicholas was nine months old, he was chosen to appear in a print ad where natural lighting was the main effect for the shot. The photo shoot was on the top floor of a rundown building that had a ceiling of windows for a natural-light effect, exactly what the ad agency wanted. However, all kinds of debris littered the stairway we had to climb to reach the photo shoot location. The place where we had to wait—I will never forget it—-was a small bedroom-sized room, containing a double bed and chairs placed next to the bed for four or five mothers and their babies and all the necessary equipment we had brought along for a day with an infant (we were told to plan on at least a couple of hours). We were cramped with nowhere for the babies to play. We had to feed them on our laps and would not dare let them down to crawl.

To make things worse, we were all told to arrive at a certain time for the shoot to begin, but when I arrived at that time the set was just being painted. Needless to say, after we had waited, whiched seemed like hours for the shoot to begin, the photographer now had cranky babies with the exception of one, and it wasn't Nicholas. The assistant to the photographer proceeded to try each child. It was a nude photo shoot of the babies, so all of the clothes had to come off each time and go back on again afterwards. We had to be ready to remove the babies' clothes on their demand. Nicholas went on camera several times with the male model, who was acting as his dad and holding him up in the air as if he were playing with his own infant. But Nicholas was not cooperating; he was tired and miserable after being cramped in close quarters for over four hours. The photographer was able to snap some pictures before Nicholas started crying, but not really enough. When Nicholas was brought back to me after the fourth try, I decided that was enough. After I dressed him and layed him on his blanket he fell fast asleep! I decided to ask the assistant on this job to sign our voucher and release us; we were going home. Was I in for a surprise! The assistant came up the stairs, wanting to try Nicholas again. She literally grabbed him off the bed and asked what right I had dressing my son without her permission! Right then and there, I told her to sign our voucher: "We are leaving; Nicholas is done for the day," I insisted. She then lectured me about my behavior and said Nicholas probably would not work in this field again, which I really didn't care; I was not going to subject my child to this dreadful situation any longer and especially not to her treatment of Nicholas. I should have left sooner. Those people did not understand how to work with children, certainly not the way other producers had in the past; nor did they have common consideration for our comfort. Nicholas was paid for the time he was at the shoot, but his photos were not used in the advertisement. And, I am happy to say, we did work in the field of modeling again.

The pictures on the next page shows what could be the nightmare of any mother whose children work in the modeling business. Nicholas was booked for a shoot for the Amway Corporation when he was six years old. We received the call on a Friday during the summer, telling us the shoot was on Monday. We had a beautiful weekend of playing out in the sun. My boys love play tattoos that wash off, and Nicholas had two tattoos on his forearm that particular weekend. Come Sunday evening when it was time to clean up for Monday morning's shoot, I removed the tattoos with soap and water. They came off, just as they usually do, but they left an imprint on Nicholas's skin from the sun. That's right! As you can see from the picture, he now had two tone images because the sun had not penetrated through the tattoos to the skin. What was I to do? It was after office hours for our talent agency, and we had to be on the set at eight o'clock Monday morning. Just to complicate the situation, he had banged his knee badly while playing as well. I decided that we should go to the shoot anyway. Not to show up at all would have been worse. Thanks to makeup that I always try to keep on hand to hide minor scrapes and small bruises, I was able to cover the tattoo markings pretty well. It was not as bad as I thought. His knee, however, was a road burn and their wasn't much I could do except keep it clean, bandage it and hope for the best. I also brought along my nephew Kenny, who is the same age as Nicholas, just in case things did not work out.

Was I surprised by the reaction of the photographer after I showed him Nicholas' knee and told him what had happened! Since I did a good job of covering up the arms, he said that was no problem. And as for the knee, "natural part of being a kid," he said. "Leave the bandage on and all. No problem!" Just when you think you have this business figured out, you don't. Often, the outcome depends on the personality of the people running the show.

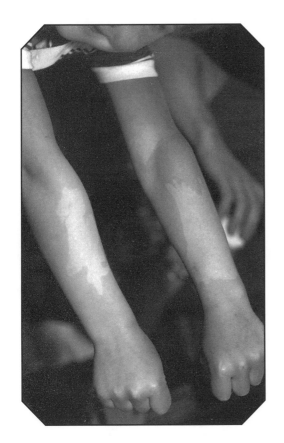

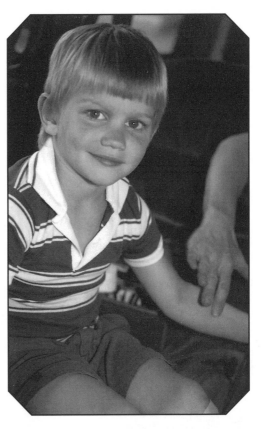

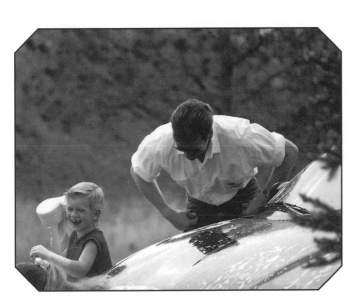

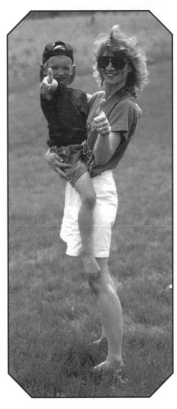

CHAPTER 7

SETTING PRIORITIES

Is This Really What You Want to Do?

Before you locate and contact agencies, sort out in your own mind whether you really want to involve your children in modeling, videos, and commercials. Try to answer these questions honestly: Does your child like people? (You don't really know until the child is a least a year old.) Are you doing it for the money? If so, think twice, because this might not be for you. You might go to audition after audition without being booked for a job. I often have been told that if you receive one job out of twelve audition calls you are not doing badly outside the larger markets! It is true that one job could end up making up for all those auditions, especially if you receive a national commercial and are booked as a principal. But such bookings might be few and far between. You have to be willing to invest some money in photographs, clothes, car expenses, and so on.

And you always have to be prepared. Do you have a flexible lifestyle? Family and friends who can help at the drop of a hat? If you have more than one child, you will need to arrange for your other children's care while you are away with one at auditions and shoots, because the others may not always be allowed to come along. Above all, if you are married, you must ask your spouse if he or she is willing to work with you and provide moral support. You will need it! Working outside of the home could present a problem, unless you prepare your employer. Sometimes, you might be given only an hour's notice to appear at an audition. Will your boss allow you to leave so suddenly? And what about school? Will your children's teachers and principals permit them to leave school to attend an audition or shoot?

Finally, are you willing to let your child be a child and have a normal, active life? For example, if while playing, your little boy or girl falls and develops a goose egg on his forehead, you might have to pass up an audition call. Worse, if he has already been chosen for an upcoming commercial but has that bump on his forehead, he probably will lose the job. But, again it depends on who is running the job. Emotionally, can you accept that potential loss?

Bumps, bruises, cuts and scrapes are all part of a young child's life. When my son Nicholas was four, he fell at preschool and lost his upper front tooth, root and all. The tooth was put back into his gum and his front teeth were wired together for four weeks. Although the gums healed and the tooth stayed in place for a while, it worked its way loose again, became infected and had to come out. In the middle of all that, Nicholas was up for a hot dog commercial. After I received the call from our talent agency that Nicholas had been tentatively booked for the commercial, I received a second call the next day requesting that I bring Nicholas to the production studio for one more look before everyone would arrive from Detroit to shoot the commercial. That tooth just didn't look right when his teeth were exposed. The last-minute look was all the director needed for him to decide not to use Nicholas. You see, he would have had to bite into a hot dog. If he had only needed to smile, he would have been fine. I will never forget how sympathetic the casting director and producer were toward us. They really wanted to use Nicholas for that shoot.

Shortly thereafter, his tooth was removed and I had to accept the fact that Nicholas would be missing that front tooth for at least three years, which would slow down his audition calls until having missing front teeth looked normal. The only considerate thing for my to do was to call all the agencies we were registered with to let them know about the situation. It was now in their hands to decide what auditions Nicholas should go on. This is another reason you do not want to spend a lot of money on professional photographs.

Over the years, I have become used to the good and the bad in this business. Most importantly, I try never to lose sight of what is in the best interest of my children. Very few children have the opportunity to experience the rewards of being in this field. While learning how to deal with many different kinds of people, my children are building self-confidence and poise. Starting as young as they did,

115

Jason and Nicholas have grown up with modeling as a natural part of their life. As long as they want to stay in this field and I am able to take them to auditions and shoots, we will continue doing it.

It is important to me as a parent as well as to them that they can play on the soccer and ice hockey teams with their friends, stay active in scouting, and participate in school-related activities. One Christmas, Nicholas played Santa Claus in his second grade school play, and nothing was going to take him away from that part. Now that the boys are older, being in this business has become their choice. They decide whether they want to go to a particular audition call or not, and they understand they cannot change their mind once they have committed themselves. Jason and Nicholas have learned that they must be responsible for their commitments in and out of the modeling industry. And I know that no one can or should force a child to perform at any age. Besides, we are a kid only once, and I don't want to push to make auditions the top priority. I want my boys to have their childhood. Too many child stars have left behind those years and can never have them back. Up to this point Jason and Nicholas have had, I feel, the best of both worlds. They have participated in a field that only a small number of other children their age have been able to experience. Right now, we are at a turning point and where the future will lead us is unknown. It is true that I am the wind beneath their wings to keep them involved, but it is also their own will that must make them want to continue to fly.

My boys might never become superstars in print or on the screen, but they will always be my superstars! Now, if you are prepared to accept the challenges I have described, let me wish you the best of luck, whatever the future may hold for you in this industry. Keeping the best interests of your family in mind, is the best advice I can give anyone who is just beginning. The family is the foundation of anyone's success. Good luck!

In the next chapter you will read about popular kids and their feelings about being in the business. These successful children could be yours or mine someday. How deeply our children become involved is up to us as their parents. It is our job to protect them and look out for their well-being.

CHAPTER 8

Sharing Thoughts of Others Growing Up in the Industry

The following excerpt is reprinted from "Her Own Person," by Jacqueling Austin, which appeared in *react magazine,* copyright 1996:

"It's way before school on a gold-green, Los Angeles day. At the Danes family's condo, early morning sun spills across white walls, a gray rug, and a litter of scripts and magazines. It's a typical day.

"In the dining room, Claire Danes' dad, Chris, pores over Web stuff on the computer, while mom Carla slaps paint on canvas. (Claire also has a brother, Asa, 22 who still lives in the family's former home base, New York City.)

"Claire, 16, comes bouncing downstairs, ready for school in navy sweats and a white t-shirt—her uniform on gym days. Her angular, red, Angela-on-*My-So-Called-Life* bob has been exchanged for a soft, sun-bleached 'do.'

"'It'—acting—is a 25-hour-a-day job. Even on this early morning, the family's phone is ringing off the hook. A famous director calls to offer a starring role in a big movie. Claire says maybe. There's a calendar on the fridge scribbled with phone numbers and question marks, with extra pieces of paper taped on and sticky notes over it all. It's a far cry from Claire's first taste of acting at 9 years old, when she was just another kid going to auditions.

"These days, Claire is in demand. She travels so much for her career that she finds being home exotic. Once home from a shoot, 'I collapse,' she says. 'No—I take off my makeup. Maybe turn on the TV and flip through channels. And do more homework. And call another friend.'

"These are long distance calls. Claire still has friends in Los Angeles from

My So-Called Life. But the ones who are from so long ago that they're family are still in New York.

"'I carry their pictures with me when I travel,' she says, explaining what seems to be the downside of being a popular, respected actress. 'I miss my friends deeply. Immensely.'"

Following is an excerpt from "Ghost of a Chance," an article written by Christine James for *BOXOFFICE* MAGAZINE (April 1995) regarding the career of fifteen-year-old Christina Ricci:

"Typecast at 15? It happens all the time on the small screen when you watch a child grow up in a role and then can't separate the person from the persona. In film, however, the audience usually get to see different facets of an actor with every part. But with Christina Ricci's dark hair, pale skin, that unsettling wisdom-beyond-her-years aura and an affinity for projects with connections to the macabre, it does seem as though a pattern is emerging.

"Ricci's credits include 'The Addams Family,' 'Addams Family Values,' and 'The Cemetery Club.' She laments that she missed out on the Kirsten Dunst role in 'Interview With the Vampire' becasue she was too old for the part, and she's currently starring in the upcoming Amblin Entertainment film adaptation of 'Casper,' the friendly ghost of Harvey Comics fame. . . .

"Ricci did . . . find out very early on that letting celebrity go to her head tended to alienate her from others her age. 'Basically, when your're a kid on a movie, and you're the only kid, everybody's going, "Oh, you're so cute, oh, you're so good, oh that was wonderful!!" like, every second. And if you believe it, and if you really allow yourself to just revel in it, and you try to go back to school, all of a sudden, people aren't telling you you're wonderful anymore. And you've still got this air like, "Wait! Aren't I wonderful?!" Then there's a problem. And I kind of went back to school after my first movie and did that for about a month, and realized, "Hey! Everyone hates me! What's up?" So I had to fix that.'

"Now, Ricci says she feels 'pretty much' like every other kid, except that she's 'really bored. I just finished working on a film ['Gaslight Addition'] and I'm at a regular high school. I've been here like a week, and I'm going out of my mind. I mean, I love working so much more.'"

118

In another article from *BOXOFFICE* MAGAZINE, "A Family Tie" (June 1995), managing editor Kim Williamson writes about the maternal side of actress Moira Kelly and the importance of her family:

"Moira Kelly believes that, in real life, being a mother is the 'role of a lifetime,' At this point in her career, the 26-year-old remains single and childless but, with her new role in 'The Tie That Blinds' Kelly can live her dream at least on the big screen. . . .

"Outside movie sets, though, her life is a different story. 'Why am I not a mom yet?' she asks rhetorically, laughing. 'It takes another partner, actually, for that to happen. This is something I like a lot of people, who are looking to get into this business to realize; It's not as easy a life as you think. It means sacrificing a lot of things like time and a settled place-especially being in my position and at my age. Still kind of starting, getting in there, proving my self. You're always moving here for three months, then here for three months. Trying to get someone to accept that—that your're going to be away for that amount of time—is hard. I don't like being away from my family and friends all the time. I don't like not being able to plan things months in advance because you don't know where you'll be. It takes a lot out of you to be in this business.'

"When she's not at work, Kelly is more than likely to be back home with her parents. 'Family is everything,' Kelly says. 'They'll accept you for anything you do. They'll love you through everything, they'll support you through everything. They'll always be there if you need them. And they're the most honest people that you'll ever come across. They'll tell you exactly what you need to know.' To repeat Moira Kelly's words, 'Family is everything.'"

To close this chapter, I offer here excerpts from "Kids," written by Liz Smith for Disney Adventures, a series of interviews with some of today's top child stars, who share thoughts regarding family, being famous, and the sacrifices that are made along the way:

"Zachery Ty Bryan, Age: 14, Claim to Fame: Plays Brad on 'Home Improvement': 'For a while, after I got the part on " H.I.," my mom and I lived in Los Angeles, and my dad and sister lived in Colorado. But it was too hard; I missed my dad so much. So then he and my sister moved out here, too. That's a dad!' Sacrifices: 'Giving up lots of time with my friends. I still have time with them, but not lots. I give up privacy. A lot of kids find out where I live and come to my house. Or if I'm playing Ding-Dong Ditchum, people can see it's me and call the *National Enquirer.* So you have to be careful. It comes with the business.'"

"Rider Strong, Age: 16, Claim to Fame: Plays Shawn on 'Boy Meets World.' Famous Face: 'I miss the anonymity of being just a regular kid. Everybody knows who I am. Kids either stalk me or they follow me and give me dirty looks because they think I'm a snob.'

"Jonathan Taylor Thomas, Age: 14, Claim to Fame: Plays Randy on 'Home Improvement,' was the voice of Simba in *The Lion King,* and played Tom Sawyer in *Tom and Huck.* Glitz and Glamour: 'When people think of Hollywood, they think, "Oh, glitz, glamour," but it's not at all like that. For Tom and Huck, we spend three months in the mud with bugs. That was a great experience, but it was tough. Then again, acting is fun, too. You get to travel to nice places and met nice people.'"

"Ben Savage, Age: 15, Claim to Fame: Plays Cory on 'Boy Meets World.' School Rules: 'I work three weeks on, one week off, usually. I attend a private school in Los Angeles. And when I'm working, I have three excellent tutors on set and I have to go to school three hours a day. Lots of kids think that's so cool—but what they don't realize is that I get home around 7 p.m. and then I have to do homework until about midnight. Then I sleep and get up at 7 a.m. It's tough because I'll go back to my regular school after having three weeks off and I'll be really far behind, or I'll come back and have to take a test that I didn't know about. I love school—my teachers at my real school are really cooperative about my schedule. I couldn't do it without them.'"

"Taran Noah Smith, Age: 11, Claim to Fame: Mark on 'Home Improvement.' Scariest Moment: 'Getting attacked by a mob of cheerleaders! My first year on "H.I.," when I was 7, I was at a Sega Kid's Star Challenge at Universal Studios, where there was a cheerleader convention. During a break, I went to Fievel's Playland. I was going down the slide when a mob a cheerleaders saw me and screamed, "It's Mark from 'Home Improvement!'" They started to climb up the slide as I was going down! I had no choice but to go through the crowd. My dad didn't stops them; he took pictures! I ran, but they were teenagers, so they caught me and grabbed my arms and legs and started swinging me. That's when a light went of in my dad's head and he realized it could be dangerous, so he stopped them!'"

And there you have it: words spoken by others who started out by auditioning for printwork, commercials, theater, or film and have become stars. Some of them started very young, like Jason and Nicholas. No one really knows what the future will bring for any of us. Let's hope that with each day we will all become better prepared to make the decisions that could possibly change our children's lives forever, and that we will keep the best interests of our entire family in mind.

GLOSSARY

Following are definitions of some of the important words one needs to know in order to function in the modeling and acting fields.

Advertisement: Pictures and/or words designed to sell a product.

AFTRA: American Federation of Television and Radio Artists, one of the theatrical unions to which a performer must belong to do live or taped TV commercials or shows.

Agency, Talent: A company that will try to promote a person in the modeling, commercial, print ad, etc. field.

Audition: To try out for a print advertisement, film, television, or stage part. Auditions are generally conducted by a casting director and/or producer.

Billboard: A large sign that advertises products or services.

Booking: To receive a job confirmation.

Call Back: An audition after a successful first audition.

Casting Director: A representative of a producer whose role is to interview and audition talent. Some production companies and ad agencies ("clients") will hire a casting director to take charge of the casting for a film or commercial. Directors work through the talent or model agency and are paid by the client. They do not receive a percentage of the performer's wages. Most casting directors keep files of talent photos and resumes.

Cattle Call: An open interview or audition at which a large number of talent shows up at the same time. No scheduled time is usually given to anyone.

Child Labor Laws: Government regulations and guidelines covering the employment of children. They vary from state to state.

Client: The company that owns the product or service to be advertised.

Composite: The calling card of the working actor and model, so to speak. An 8" x 10" sheet printed on one or two sides with photos of the talent, in a variety of formats, and color or black and white. It is sent to a talent agency, which in turn sends it to the casting people and is also given out by the performer at auditions, casting calls, etc.

Contact Sheet: A photographic print sheet made up of all the shots from a roll of film, used to determine which photos are to be enlarged.

Day Rate: Compensation paid to talent for the day only and usually without further compensation.

Exclusive: Being listed with only one talent agency at a time and for a specific length of time.

Extra: A person hired usually to be in a group of people and not seen up front and center in the camera.

Go-See: An audition to see if a studio wants to hire a model, usually for print.

Headshot: One photo of person's head from the shoulders up.

Holding Fee: The amount of money paid to an actor every thirteen weeks for as long as a commercial is being held by an ad agency. The fee is generally the same as the original session fee.

Iced: To be on-hold for a particular booking for which one auditioned.

Industrial: A filmed or live production used for promotion. It may be an educational, sales, or instructional film, but not a commercial film meant for general release.

Letter of Intent: Letter from the talent agency stating it intends to attempt to secure employment for talent as an actor/model and conform with the relevant child labor laws.

Location: A place away from the studio to which one travels for a booking.

Look-See: Same as "audition" and "go-see."

Multi-Listed: Registered with more than one talent agency.

National: Advertising that might be seen anywhere in the United States.

Non-SAG: A production which occurs without the sanction of SAG; union members may not appear in this type of production.

Product Packaging: A person's photograph appears directly on the product box, bottle, etc.

Point of Purchase: A person's photograph appears near where a product is being sold, but not directly on the product itself.

Principal: A person who is usually up front on a camera shoot and may or may not have spoken lines and who is usually paid more than an extra.

Print Work: Photos in printed materials, such as publications, packaging, posters, etc.

Producer: The person responsible for making decisions on a production.

Production Company: A firm that makes television commercials, industrial videos, educational, information films, full-length movies, etc.

Product Conflict: Appearing in one commercial and then auditioning for the competitor's product within a certain length of time.

Proofs: Pictures from a still photo shooting from which a selection can be made for the final print(s).

Rate: The amount of money per hour a performer or model receives for services. A day rate is the charge for a whole day. A model might be booked for a weekly rate or an overall job rate.

Regional: Advertising limited to a region. Usually a region is divided, for example: North Central, Northwest, South Central, Southeast, Southwest, and West Coast.

Residual: The fee paid for each broadcast of a commercial after the initial airing. The amount varies depending upon how many times, over what length of time and in what markets the commercial is shown. Also the size of the the performer's roll is a factor to determine the residual rate.

Resume: A listing of all jobs one has had in the industry, and vital statistics. It usually is attached to a photo or composite.

Screen Actors Guild (SAG): The union a performer must belong to in order to do films, whether for motion pictures or television provided the producer or distributor is a signatory to the SAG agreement. Tape, used in television broadcast, is covered by AFTRA.

Session Fee: Performance pay for a single airing of a commercial.

Stand-In: A substitute for featured talent, used for light setting, placements, etc.

Statistics: Information about a person listed on the composite or resume; such as age, clothing size, height, weight, measurements, hair coloring, eye color. Some include special abilities for example, singing, dancing, etc.

Story Board: A copy of audition lines with cartoon-like pictures showing examples of what the actor should do for the audition.

Taft-Hartley Law: A Federal law providing that a person can work a certain amount of time on a union job without having to join that union. An actor can work up to thirty calendar days of a first job without being required to join the union. On the second job, or any job obtained after thirty calendar days, or any job that lasts over thirty calendar days, one must join the appropriate union.

Talent: A person or people chosen to appear in a print advertisement, commercial, or video.

Tear Sheets: Pages from a publication in which a model has appeared.

Test Commercial: A commercial scheduled to be aired in a small area and monitored for its effectiveness.

Voice-Over: The sound from the announcer or even the pictured actor during the running of the commercial. Someone might be hired to do the voice if the talent doing the acting is not good at speaking lines or if a particular voice is desired.

Voucher: A form from the talent agency that is filled out and signed by the talent and representative on the job location. It includes the talent's name, the client, product, to and from times, and all rates that apply at the time.

Wild Spot: A commercial that runs on a non-network or independent station, or a spot that runs between scheduled off network programming.

Work Permit: A form giving a person under age 18 permission to work during certain hours and under certain conditions.

AFTERWORD

Before I go, I must say, THANK YOU. I hope that your purchase of this book proves to be a good investment for you. Your purchase will also help others, such as *The Children's Miracle Network Telethon,* which was started by the Osmond Family. A portion of the profits from this book will be donated to that charity.

CHECKLIST

1. After reading this book, you have analyzed your situation and decided to try modeling.

2. Chose the regional SAG office closest to your home and call to make sure it is still located at the address listed in this book. Chapter 2

3. Send for the list of agencies and include a self-addressed stamped envelope for faster return of materials.

4. While waiting for the list of agencies, take your own snapshots and have them developed. Chapter 3

5. When the list arrives, chose three to five agencies or more if you perfer, and call them to verfiy their procedures and addresses and that they register children the ages of yours.

6. Follow the agencies' instructions for registering. Send them photos and statistics of your child. Obtain a work permit and social security number (if you have not already done so) for your child. Chapter 2

7. Wait for audition calls. In the meantime, make sure you have someone to call, should you need a last-minute babysitter for your other children.

8. When the call comes, write down everything, including directions and dates. Remember to keep a note pad and pencil by your phones. Cross check the date of the audition and shoot on your calendar and with your family. See page 133.

9. Map your route; bring appropriate drinks, snacks, entertainment for your child's age; go to the audition. Wait for the agency's call. If no call, let it go!

10. When an agency calls to say that you received the job, note exact dates, time, and location of shoot, as well as clothing requirements, etc.

11. Map your route, if different from the audition. Once again pack your bag of necessities for the day. Go to the shoot. Chapter 5

12. Have necessary paperwork filled out at job and signed. Mail one copy to agency with self-addressed stamped envelope as soon as possible to receive payment of a non-union job. Keep one copy for your records. If more than four weeks pass, make a follow-up call to the agency. Chapter 5

BIBLIOGRAPHY

Ross Reports Television, Television Index, Inc., 40-29 27th Street, Long Island City, N.Y. 11101. (718) 937-3990

CD Directory, Breakdown Services, LTD., 1120 S. Robertson, 3rd Floor, Los Angeles, CA 90035. (310) 276-9166

Casting Society of America, 311 West 43rd Street, New York, New York 10036. (212) 333-4552

BOXOFFICE Magazine, 6640 Sunset Blvd., Suite 100, Hollywood, CA 90028 or 819 South Wabash Ave., Chicago, IL 60605

ABC Pictures, Inc., 1867 E. Florida, Springfield, MO 65803. (417) 869-3456. To request a catalog of services for modeling composites, etc.

Disney Adventures, P.O Box 420200, Palm Coast, Florida 32142-0200. (800) 829-5146

react magazine, Advance Magazine Publications, Inc., 711 Third Avenue, New York, NY 10017. (212) 450-0921

TELEVISION INDEX INFORMATION SERVICES include a group of weekly reports - plus a semi-annual index covering network television programming, advertising, production activities and performances, supported by a subscribers information service. **Television Index** began reporting and recording network, syndicated and special television program activities in 1949, and the records are always open to subscribers, who may call or write at any time for information, without charge. Special research services are available only to subscribers. **Television Index** publications are available by subscription in combinations and individually as noted in the subscription form at the bottom of the page.

TELEVISION INDEX (*Weekly*). The Network Program Report covers all commercial network series debuting or returning during the current week, with production credits, and history; also all network specials in each week, including variety shows and documentaries, with credits and sponsors. The Public Affairs section produces a continuing record of guest and subjects of news, public affairs, religious and sports programs. The Program Performance Record provides writer, director, performer and other production credits for the week's network programs that involve changing or guest dramatic or variety performers or talk show guests. Theatrical and made-for-TV movies are designated in the listings and each week's reports indicates the number of original episodes of each series that have been presented during the season. The Production Register contains a yearly report of network program production information, including reports on major studios and major independent television production organizations and the production divisions of the four networks. The sevice has a semi-annual cumulative index to the Network Program Report.

TV PRO-LOG (*Weekly*). Newsletter of information and comment about and on the current production scene. Each week, the newsletter reports the present and future of television production and program activities, including movements of key production personnel, concisely and authoritatively, for the television professional.

NETWORK FUTURES (*Weekly*). Calendar-guide listings for upcoming series, debuts, returns, program specials and schedule changes. Each newsletter lists brief details in the network picture, including stars, sponsors and major production people concerned with new and returning series and special programs.

ROSS REPORTS RADIO-TV CONTACT SERVICE (*Quarterly*). Directory to radio and television news and talk shows in the New York City area, including network and syndicated talk shows. Published February, May, August & November. Over 50 pages, 4 x 6 1/2 inches. Paper Cover.

ROSS REPORTS TELEVISION (*Monthly*). Directory, production and casting guide, designed for actors and writers, with production personnel concerned with all network series. The directory lists New York advertising agencies with in-house casting departments, casting directors, franchised talent agents, literary agents, commercial producers, network program packagers, network production and casting information for New York-originating programs, and production, script and casting information for primetime series and daytime dramas in Los Angeles and New York. Each issue is an update of the previous month's issue, published during the first week of each month. Over 60 pages, 4 x 6 1/2 inches, including TV Pro-Log Digest.

ROSS REPORTS, U.S.A. (*Quarterly*). Directory designed for actors listing franchised talent agents around the country, exclusive of New York, and Personal Managers throughout the country, including New York, who are members of the National Conference of Personal Managers or the Conference of Personal Managers. Published February, May, August & November. Over 60 pages, 4 x 6 1/2 inches. Paper Cover.

TELEVISION INDEX ANNUAL (*Annual*). Each report lists the past season's commercial network primetime programs in detail including packager and producer, brief description of the show with cast, production credits and a history of the series. The annual also includes a list of network pilots, reality-based series, theatrical films, made-for-television movies and mini-series that debuted during the season. The first issue covered the 1989-90 television season.

WRITERS DIRECTORY/PRODUCTION REGISTER (*Annual*). Seasonal listing of writers for series, movies and specials with series, episode title and original air date. Seasonal listing of network program packagers and the series, pilots, movies, variety shows and entertainment specials they produced during the season. The first issue covered the 1991-92 season.

————————————————— CUT HERE —————————————————

Subscriptions to Television Index Services and Publications	Annual Fee
___ **TELEVISION INDEX Information Service,** with Network Program Report, TV Pro-Log, Network Futures, Cumulative Index, Production Register, Television Annual, unlimited information service	$250.00
___ **TELEVISION INDEX Information Services,** same publications included as above; *special rate for University/College Libraries and Municipal Public Libraries Only*	$165.00
___ **TELEVISION ANNUAL,** for each television season, September through August (published in December), complete information for the preceding television season	$10.00
___ **WRITERS DIRECTORY/PRODUCTION REGISTER,** for each television season, September through August (published in October),	$20.00
___ **TV PRO-LOG** (*Weekly*), newsletter on present and future television production **in combination with** **NETWORK FUTURES** (*Weekly*), calender guide to upcoming programming.	$100.0C
___ **ROSS REPORTS TELEVISION** (*Monthly*), New York casting and national production guide (Separate from Television Index Service Subscription)	MUST BE PREPAID $42.75
___ **ROSS REPORTS USA** (*Quarterly*), Available in single copy only (Separate from Television Index Service Subscription)	MUST BE PREPAID $5.70
___ **ROSS REPORTS RADIO-TV CONTACT SERVICE** (*Quarterly*), Available in single copy only (Separate from Television Index Service Subscription)	MUST BE PREPAID $5.70

(Add 8 1/4% New York Sales Tax for all New York residents)

Name——————————————————— Title ——————————— ——Check Enclosed

Organization ———————————————————————————— ——Bill Organization

Address———————————————————————————— ___Bill Me

City ——————————State ——————————— Zip Code———————

——————————————
Authorization Signature

TELEVISION INDEX, INC.   40-29 27th Street   Long Island City,   New York 11101   (718) 937-3990

Talent Agency Contact List

1) _____

_____

_____

2) _____

_____

_____

3) _____

_____

_____

4) _____

_____

_____

5) _____

_____

_____

6) _____

_____

_____

7) _____

_____

_____

Audition Call / Job Information Sheet

Date of Call: _____

Agency That Called: _____

Time of Audition: _____

Date of Audition: _____

Location: _____

Directions: _____

_____

Contact Person (and phone number if available): _____

Type of Audition: (Print, Commercial, Nat'l, Regional, Union or Non-Union, Etc.)

_____

Rate (if known): _____

Type of Clothes to Wear: _____

Call Back Date _____

Actual Shoot Date: _____

Received Job?:   YES   NO

If yes, you should ask many of the same questions as above.

Shoot Date: _____

Time: _____

Location (if different than audition): _____

_____

Contact Person (and phone number if available): _____

Clothes, Props Needed by Talent: _____

Vouchers: Make sure to know who has vouchers that must be filled out.

CALLING ALL READERS

Now, if you are willing, it is time for you to write to me and let me know your thoughts regarding the book. Did it lead you to the least expensive way to register your children with talent agencies? Did it give you an insight into the industry and show you what to expect? I would appreciate receiving comments from readers about how this book helped you. Please indicate whether I may quote you or use your name in my newsletter. Mark you envelope "Readers' Comments." Thank you in advance for your valuable response.

Send your comments to:
> Believe in Yourself Publishing Co.
> P.O. Box 89
> Fruitport, MI 49415

NEWSLETTER ORDER FORM

THE CLAPBOARD NEWS

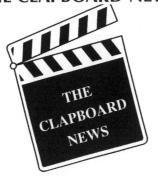

January, April, July, and October

- The quarterly Newsletter will keep you updated about the latest name and address changes in the industry.

- Learn about auditions in several area cities; and at Walt Disney Theme Parks, Opryland USA Productions, and others.

- Listen to the industry talk to you.

- This is where I want to hear from you, the reader, regarding how this book helped you get started. Share your child's first audition or job experience with all of us.

- In the question and answer section, we can help each other. You can have your questions answered and learn from others' queries.

Please send your name and address, plus a check or money order (no cash or COD) for $8.95 (MI residents add 6% sales tax) for a year's subscription to the quarterly Newsletter to: Believe in Yourself Publishing Co., P.O. Box 89, Fruitport, Michigan 49415. Please mark envelope "Newsletter Subscription."

Allow four to six weeks for delivery of first newsletter.

Index

JASON AND NICHOLAS,

YOUR GREATEST ROLL OF ALL:

JUST BEING A KID, A FRIEND,

A SON,

AND A BROTHER,

AN EXCITING LIFE WITH ONE PROUD

FATHER AND MOTHER

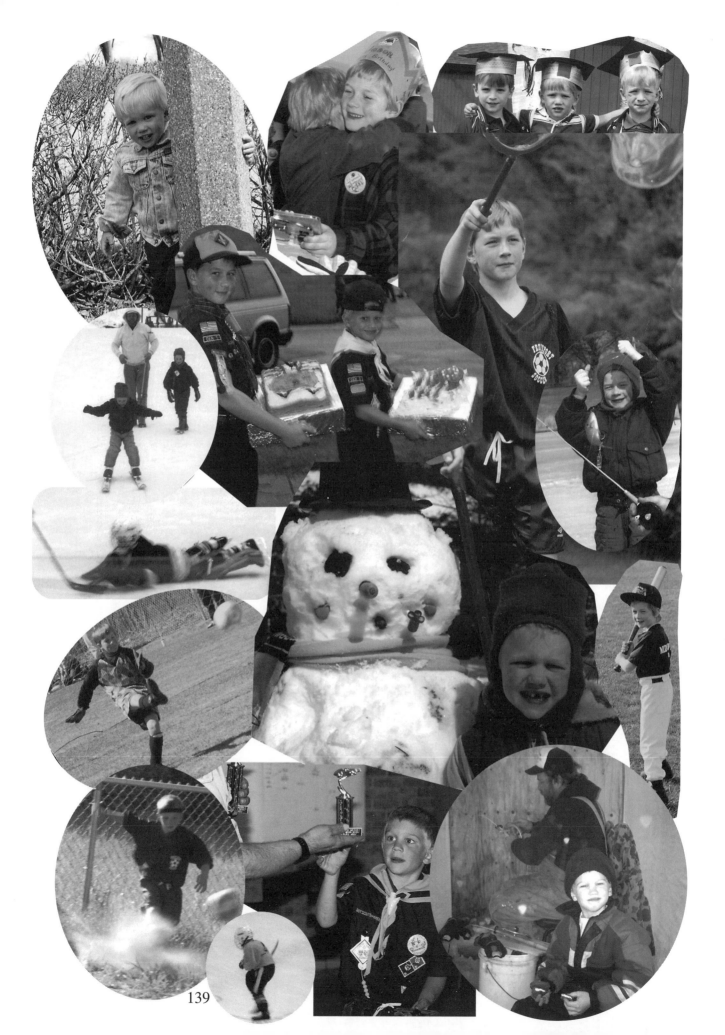

139

BOOK ORDER FORM

To Give to a Friend or Relative
(Makes a great gift)

Send check or money order (no cash or COD) for $29.95 + $3.99 for shipping and handling to: Believe in Yourself Publishing Co., P.O. Box 89, Fruitport, Michigan 49415. Michigan residents add 6% sales tax. Please mark envelope, "Book Order."

Allow four to six weeks for delivery.

OR

For faster delivery, order by phone with your American Express, Visa or Master Card: 1-800-873-0653.

- Tear along dotted line -

Name: _____

Address: _____

_____

Number of books ordered: _____

X $33.94 (MI residents add 6% sales tax)

for each book ordered = _____

Amount of check or money order enclosed _____

NOTES

NOTES